GUIDELINES FOR THE SAFE USE OF
WASTEWATER, EXCRETA AND GREYWATER

Volume 2
Wastewater use in agriculture

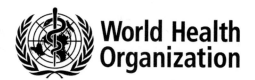
World Health Organization

WHO Library Cataloguing-in-Publication Data

WHO guidelines for the safe use of wastewater, excreta and greywater / World Health Organization.

v. 1. Policy and regulatory aspects — v. 2. Wastewater use in agriculture — v. 3. Wastewater and excreta use in aquaculture — v. 4. Excreta and greywater use in agriculture.

1. Water supply. 2. Water supply - legislation. 3. Agriculture. 4. Aquaculture. 5. Sewage. 6. Wastewater treatment plants. 7. Guidelines. I. World Health Organization. II. Title: Safe use of wastewater, excreta and greywater. III. Title: Policy and regulatory aspects. IV. Title: Wastewater use in agriculture. V. Title: Wastewater and excreta use in aquaculture. VI. Title: Excreta and greywater use in agriculture.

ISBN 92 4 154686 7 (set)   (NLM classification: WA 675)
ISBN 92 4 154682 4 (v. 1)
ISBN 92 4 154683 2 (v. 2)
ISBN 92 4 154684 0 (v. 3)
ISBN 92 4 154685 9 (v. 4)

CONTENTS

LIST OF ACRONYMS AND ABBREVIATIONS

ADI	acceptable daily intake
BOD	biochemical oxygen demand
2,4-D	2,4-dichlorophenoxyacetic acid
DALY	disability adjusted life year
DDT	dichlorodiphenyltrichloroethane
EC_{DW}	electrical conductivity of the drainage water
EC_W	electrical conductivity of the irrigation water
FAO	Food and Agriculture Organization of the United Nations
HIA	health impact assessment
ID_{50}	median infective dose
LF	leaching fraction
MDG	Millennium Development Goal
NOAEL	no-observed-adverse-effect level
OR	odds ratio
PAH	polycyclic aromatic hydrocarbon
PCB	polychlorinated biphenyl
PPPY	per person per year
QMRA	quantitative microbial risk assessment
SAR	sodium adsorption ratio
SAT	soil aquifer treatment
2,4,5-T	2,4,5-trichlorophenoxyacetic acid
TC	total coliforms
TDI	tolerable daily intake
TDS	total dissolved solids
TN	total nitrogen
TOC	total organic carbon
TSS	total suspended solids
UASB	upflow anaerobic sludge blanket
WHO	World Health Organization
WTO	World Trade Organization

PREFACE

The United Nations General Assembly (2000) adopted the Millennium Development Goals (MDGs) on 8 September 2000. The MDGs that are most directly related to the use of wastewater in agriculture are "Goal 1: Eliminate extreme poverty and hunger" and "Goal 7: Ensure environmental sustainability." The use of wastewater in agriculture can help communities to grow more food and make use of precious water and nutrient resources. However, it should be done safely to maximize public health gains and environmental benefits.

To protect public health and facilitate the rational use of wastewater and excreta in agriculture and aquaculture, in 1973, the World Health Organization (WHO) developed guidelines for wastewater use in agriculture and aquaculture under the title *Reuse of effluents: Methods of wastewater treatment and health safeguards* (WHO, 1973). After a thorough review of epidemiological studies and other information, the guidelines were updated in 1989 as *Health guidelines for the use of wastewater in agriculture and aquaculture* (WHO, 1989). These guidelines have been very influential, and many countries have adopted or adapted them for their wastewater and excreta use practices.

Wastewater use in agriculture is increasingly considered a method combining water and nutrient recycling, increased household food security and improved nutrition for poor households. Interest in wastewater use in agriculture has been driven by water scarcity, lack of availability of nutrients and concerns about health and environmental effects. It was necessary to update the guidelines to take into account recent scientific evidence concerning pathogens, chemicals and other factors, including changes in population characteristics, changes in sanitation practices, better methods for evaluating risk, social/equity issues and sociocultural practices. There was a particular need to conduct a review of both risk assessment and epidemiological data.

In order to better package the guidelines for appropriate audiences, the third edition of the *Guidelines for the safe use of wastewater, excreta and greywater* is presented in four separate volumes: *Volume 1: Policy and regulatory aspects*; *Volume 2: Wastewater use in agriculture*; *Volume 3: Wastewater and excreta use in aquaculture*; and *Volume 4: Excreta and greywater use in agriculture*.

WHO water-related guidelines are based on scientific consensus and best available evidence and are developed through broad participation. The *Guidelines for the safe use of wastewater, excreta and greywater* are designed to protect the health of farmers (and their families), local communities and product consumers. They are meant to be adapted to take into consideration national, sociocultural, economic and environmental factors. Where the Guidelines relate to technical issues — for example, wastewater treatment — technologies that are readily available and achievable (from both technical and economic standpoints) are explicitly noted, but others are not excluded. Overly strict standards may not be sustainable and, paradoxically, may lead to reduced health protection, because they may be viewed as unachievable under local circumstances and, thus, ignored. The Guidelines therefore strive to maximize overall public health benefits and the beneficial use of scarce resources.

Following an expert meeting in Stockholm, Sweden, WHO published *Water quality: Guidelines, standards and health — Assessment of risk and risk management for water-related infectious disease* (Fewtrell & Bartram, 2001). This document presents a harmonized framework for the development of guidelines and standards for water-related microbial hazards. This framework involves the assessment of health risks prior to the setting of health targets, defining basic control approaches and evaluating the impact of these combined approaches on public health status. The framework is flexible and allows countries to take into consideration associated health risks that may result from microbial exposures through drinking-water or contact with recreational or occupational water. It is important that health risks from the use of wastewater in agriculture be put into the context of the overall level of disease within a given population.

This volume of the *Guidelines for the safe use of wastewater, excreta and greywater* provides information on the assessment and management of risks associated with microbial hazards and toxic chemicals. It explains requirements to promote the safe use of wastewater in agriculture, including minimum procedures and specific health-based targets, and how those requirements are intended to be used. This volume also describes the approaches used in deriving the guidelines, including health-based targets, and includes a substantive revision of approaches to ensuring microbial safety.

This edition of the Guidelines supersedes previous editions (1973 and 1989). The Guidelines are recognized as representing the position of the United Nations system on issues of wastewater, excreta and greywater use and health by "UN-Water," the coordinating body of the 24 United Nations agencies and programmes concerned with water issues. This edition of the Guidelines further develops concepts, approaches and information in previous editions and includes additional information on:

- the context of overall waterborne disease burden in a population and how the use of wastewater in agriculture may contribute to that burden;
- the Stockholm Framework for development of water-related guidelines and the setting of health-based targets;
- risk analysis;
- risk management strategies, including quantification of different health protection measures;
- chemicals;
- guideline implementation strategies.

The revised Guidelines will be useful to all those concerned with issues relating to the safe use of wastewater, excreta and greywater, public health and water and waste management, including environmental and public health scientists, educators, researchers, engineers, policy-makers and those responsible for developing standards and regulations.

ACKNOWLEDGEMENTS

The World Health Organization (WHO) wishes to express its appreciation to all those whose efforts made possible the production of the *Guidelines for the safe use of wastewater, excreta and greywater, Volume 2: Wastewater use in agriculture*, in particular Dr Jamie Bartram (Coordinator, Water, Sanitation and Health, WHO, Geneva) and Mr Richard Carr (Technical Officer, Water, Sanitation and Health, WHO, Geneva), who coordinated the development of the Guidelines.

An international group of experts provided material and participated in the development and review of Volume 2 of the *Guidelines for the safe use of wastewater, excreta and greywater*. Many individuals contributed to each chapter, directly and through associated activities. The contributions[1] of the following individuals to the development of these Guidelines are appreciated:

Mohammad Abed Aziz Al-Rasheed, Ministry of Health, Amman, Jordan

Saqer Al Salem, WHO Regional Centre for Environmental Health Activities, Amman, Jordan

John Anderson, New South Wales Department of Public Works & Services, Sydney, Australia

Andreas Angelakis, National Foundation for Agricultural Research, Institute of Iraklio, Iraklio, Greece

Takashi Asano,* University of California at Davis, Davis, California, USA

Nicholas Ashbolt,* University of New South Wales, Sydney, Australia

Lorimer Mark Austin, Council for Scientific and Industrial Research, Pretoria, South Africa

Ali Akbar Azimi, University of Tehran, Tehran, Iran

Javed Aziz, University of Engineering & Technology, Lahore, Pakistan

Akiça Bahri, National Research Institute for Agricultural Engineering, Water, and Forestry, Ariana, Tunisia

Mohamed Bazza, Food and Agriculture Organization of the United Nations, Cairo, Egypt

Ursula Blumenthal,* London School of Hygiene and Tropical Medicine, London, United Kingdom

Jean Bontoux, University of Montpellier, Montpellier, France

Laurent Bontoux, European Commission, Brussels, Belgium

Robert Bos, WHO, Geneva, Switzerland

François Brissaud, University of Montpellier II, Montpellier, France

Stephanie Buechler,* International Water Management Institute, Pantancheru, Andhra Pradesh, India

Paulina Cervantes-Olivier, French Environmental Health Agency, Maisons Alfort, France

Andrew Chang,* University of California at Riverside, Riverside, California, USA

Guéladio Cissé, Swiss Centre for Scientific Research, Abidjan, Côte d'Ivoire

Joseph Cotruvo, J. Cotruvo & Associates, Washington, DC, USA

Brian Crathorne, RWE Thames Water, Reading, United Kingdom

David Cunliffe, Environmental Health Service, Adelaide, Australia

---

[1] An asterisk (*) indicates the preparation of substantial text inputs.

Anders Dalsgaard,* Royal Veterinary and Agricultural University, Frederiksberg, Denmark

Gayathri Devi,* International Water Management Institute, Pantancheru, Andhra Pradesh, India

Pay Drechsel, International Water Management Institute, Accra, Ghana

Bruce Durham, Veolia Water Systems, Derbyshire, United Kingdom

Peter Edwards,* Asian Institute of Technology, Klong Luang, Thailand

Dirk Engels, WHO, Geneva, Switzerland

Badri Fattel, The Hebrew University Jerusalem, Jerusalem, Israel

John Fawell, independent consultant, Flackwell Heath, United Kingdom

Pinchas Fine, Institute of Soil, Water and Environmental Sciences, Bet-Dagan, Israel

Jay Fleisher, Nova Southeastern University, Fort Lauderdale, Florida, USA

Yanfen Fu, National Centre for Rural Water Supply Technical Guidance, Beijing, People's Republic of China

Yaya Ganou, Ministry of Health, Ouagadougou, Burkina Faso

Alan Godfrey, United Utilities Water, Warrington, United Kingdom

Maria Isabel Gonzalez Gonzalez, National Institute of Hygiene, Epidemiology and Microbiology, Havana, Cuba

Cagatay Guler, Hacettepe University, Ankara, Turkey

Gary Hartz, Director, Indian Health Service, Rockville, Maryland, USA

Paul Heaton, Power and Water Corporation, Darwin, Northern Territory, Australia

Ivanildo Hespanhol, University of Sao Paolo, Sao Paolo, Brazil

Jose Hueb, WHO, Geneva, Switzerland

Petter Jenssen,* University of Life Sciences, Aas, Norway

Blanca Jiménez,* National Autonomous University of Mexico, Mexico City, Mexico

Jean-François Junger, European Commission, Brussels, Belgium

Ioannis K. Kalavrouziotis, University of Ioannina, Agrinio, Greece

Peter Kolsky, World Bank, Washington, DC, USA

Doulaye Koné,* Swiss Federal Institute for Environmental Science and Technology (EAWAG) / Department of Water and Sanitation in Developing Countries (SANDEC), Duebendorf, Switzerland

Sasha Koo-Oshima, Food and Agriculture Organization of the United Nations, Rome, Italy

Alice Sipiyian Lakati, Department of Environmental Health, Nairobi, Kenya

Valentina Lazarova, ONDEO Services, Le Pecq, France

Pascal Magoarou, European Commission, Brussels, Belgium

Duncan Mara,* University of Leeds, Leeds, United Kingdom

Gerardo Mogol, Department of Health, Manila, Philippines

Gerald Moy, WHO, Geneva, Switzerland

Rafael Mujeriego, Technical University of Catalonia, Barcelona, Spain

Constantino Nurizzo, Politecnico di Milano, Milan, Italy

Gideon Oron, Ben-Gurion University of the Negev, Kiryat Sde-Boker, Israel

Mohamed Ouahdi, Ministry of Health and Population, Algiers, Algeria

Albert Page,* University of California at Riverside, Riverside, California, USA

Genxing Pan,* Nanjing Agricultural University, Nanjing, People's Republic of China

Nikolaos Paranychianakis, National Foundation for Agricultural Research, Institute of Iraklio, Iraklio, Greece

Martin Parkes, North China College of Water Conservancy and Hydropower, Zhengzhou, Henan, People's Republic of China

Anne Peasey,* Imperial College (formerly with London School of Hygiene and Tropical Medicine), London, United Kingdom

Susan Petterson,* University of New South Wales, Sydney, Australia

Liqa Raschid-Sally, International Water Management Institute, Accra, Ghana

Kerstin Röske, Institute for Medicine, Microbiology and Hygiene, Dresden, Germany

Lorenzo Savioli, WHO, Geneva, Switzerland

Caroline Schönning, Swedish Institute for Infectious Disease Control, Stockholm, Sweden

Janine Schwartzbrod, University of Nancy, Nancy, France

Louis Schwartzbrod, University of Nancy, Nancy, France

Jørgen Schlundt, WHO, Geneva, Switzerland

Natalia Shapirova, Ministry of Health, Tashkent, Uzbekistan

Hillel Shuval, The Hebrew University of Jerusalem, Jerusalem, Israel

Thor-Axel Stenström,* Swedish Institute for Infectious Disease Control, Stockholm, Sweden

Martin Strauss,* Swiss Federal Institute for Environmental Science and Technology (EAWAG) / Department of Water and Sanitation in Developing Countries (SANDEC), Duebendorf, Switzerland

Ted Thairs, EUREAU Working Group on Wastewater Reuse (former Secretary), Herefordshire, United Kingdom

Terrence Thompson, WHO Regional Office for the Western Pacific, Manila, Philippines

Sarah Tibatemwa, National Water & Sewerage Corporation, Kampala, Uganda

Andrea Tilche, European Commission, Brussels, Belgium

Mwakio P. Tole, Kenyatta University, Nairobi, Kenya

Francisco Torrella, University of Murcia, Murcia, Spain

Hajime Toyofuku, WHO, Geneva, Switzerland

Wim van der Hoek, independent consultant, Landsmeer, The Netherlands

Johan Verink, ICY Waste Water & Energy, Hanover, Germany

Marcos von Sperling, Federal University of Minas Gerais, Belo Horizonte, Brazil

Christine Werner, Deutsche Gesellschaft für Technische Zusammenarbeit (GTZ), Eschborn, Germany

Steve White, RWE Thames Water, Reading, United Kingdom

Thanks are also due to Marla Sheffer for editing the complete text of the Guidelines, Windy Prohom and Colette Desigaud for their assistance in project administration and Peter Gosling, who acted as the rapporteur for the Final Review Meeting for the Finalization of the Third Edition of the WHO Guidelines for the Safe Use of Wastewater, Excreta and Greywater in Geneva.

The preparation of these Guidelines would not have been possible without the generous support of the United Kingdom Department for International Development, the Swedish International Development Cooperation Agency (Sida), partly through the Stockholm Environment Institute, the Norwegian Ministry of Foreign Affairs, the German Gesellschaft für Technische Zusammenarbeit GmbH and the Dutch Ministry of Foreign Affairs (DGIS) through WASTE (Advisors on Urban Environment and Development).

EXECUTIVE SUMMARY

This volume of the World Health Organization's (WHO) *Guidelines for the safe use of wastewater, excreta and greywater* describes the present state of knowledge regarding the impact of wastewater use in agriculture on the health of product consumers, workers and their families and local communities. Health hazards are identified for each vulnerable group, and appropriate health protection measures to mitigate the risks are discussed.

The primary aim of the Guidelines is to maximize public health protection and the beneficial use of important resources. The purpose of this volume of the Guidelines is to ensure that the use of wastewater in agriculture is made as safe as possible, so that the nutritional and household food security benefits can be shared widely within communities whose livelihood depends on wastewater-irrigated agriculture. Thus, the adverse health impacts of wastewater use in agriculture should be carefully weighed against the benefits to health and the environment associated with these practices. Yet this is not a matter of simple trade-offs. Wherever wastewater use in agriculture contributes significantly to food security and nutritional status, the point is to identify associated hazards, define the risks they represent to vulnerable groups and design measures aimed at reducing these risks.

This volume of the Guidelines is intended to be used as the basis for the development of international and national approaches (including standards and regulations) to managing the health risks from hazards associated with wastewater use in agriculture, as well as providing a framework for national and local decision-making. The information provided is applicable to the intentional use of wastewater in agriculture and is also relevant where faecally contaminated water is used for irrigation unintentionally.

The Guidelines provide an integrated preventive management framework for safety applied from the point of wastewater generation to the consumption of products grown with the wastewater and excreta. They describe reasonable minimum requirements of good practice to protect the health of the people using wastewater or excreta or consuming products grown with wastewater or excreta and provide information that is then used to derive health-based targets. Neither the minimum good practices nor the health-based targets are mandatory limits. The preferred approaches adopted by national or local authorities towards implementation of the Guidelines, including health-based targets, may vary depending on local social, cultural, environmental and economic conditions, as well as knowledge of routes of exposure, the nature and severity of hazards and the effectiveness of health protection measures available.

The revised *Guidelines for the safe use of wastewater, excreta and greywater* will be useful to all those concerned with issues relating to the safe use of wastewater, excreta and greywater, public health, water resources development and wastewater management. The target audience may include public health, agricultural and environmental scientists, agriculture professionals, educators, researchers, engineers, policy-makers and those responsible for developing standards and regulations.

Introduction

Wastewater is increasingly used for agriculture in both developing and industrialized countries, and the principal driving forces are:

- increasing water scarcity and stress, and degradation of freshwater resources resulting from improper disposal of wastewater;
- population increase and related increased demand for food and fibre;
- a growing recognition of the resource value of wastewater and the nutrients it contains;
- the Millennium Development Goals (MDGs), especially the goals for ensuring environmental sustainability and eliminating poverty and hunger.

It is estimated that, within the next 50 years, more than 40% of the world's population will live in countries facing water stress or water scarcity (Hinrichsen, Robey & Upadhyay, 1998). Growing competition between the agricultural and urban uses of high-quality freshwater supplies, particularly in arid, semi-arid and densely populated regions, will increase the pressure on this ever scarcer resource.

Most population growth is expected to occur in urban and periurban areas in developing countries (United Nations Population Division, 2002). Population growth increases both the demand for fresh water and the amount of wastes that are discharged into the environment, thus leading to more pollution of clean water sources.

Wastewater is often a reliable year-round source of water, and it contains the nutrients necessary for plant growth. The value of wastewater has long been recognized by farmers worldwide. The use of wastewater in agriculture is a form of nutrient and water recycling, and this often reduces downstream environmental impacts on soil and water resources.

The United Nations General Assembly adopted the MDGs on 8 September 2000 (United Nations General Assembly, 2000). The MDGs most directly related to the use of wastewater in agriculture are "Goal 1: Eliminate extreme poverty and hunger" and "Goal 7: Ensure environmental sustainability." The use of wastewater in agriculture can help communities to grow more food and conserve precious water and nutrient resources.

The Stockholm Framework

The Stockholm Framework is an integrated approach that combines risk assessment and risk management to control water-related diseases. This provides a harmonized framework for the development of health-based guidelines and standards in terms of water- and sanitation-related microbial hazards. The Stockholm Framework involves the assessment of health risks prior to the setting of health-based targets and the development of guideline values, defining basic control approaches and evaluating the impact of these combined approaches on public health. The Stockholm Framework provides the conceptual framework for these Guidelines and other WHO water-related guidelines.

Assessment of health risk

Three types of evaluations are used to assess risk: microbial and chemical laboratory analysis, epidemiological studies and quantitative microbial (and chemical) risk assessment.

Wastewater contains a variety of different pathogens, many of which are capable of survival in the environment (in the wastewater, on the crops or in the soil) long enough to be transmitted to humans. Table 1 presents a summary of the information available from epidemiological studies of infectious disease transmission related to

Table 1. Summary of health risks associated with the use of wastewater for irrigation

Group exposed	Health risks		
	Helminth infections	**Bacterial/virus infections**	**Protozoal infections**
Consumers	Significant risk of *Ascaris* infection for both adults and children with untreated wastewater	Cholera, typhoid and shigellosis outbreaks reported from use of untreated wastewater; seropositive responses for *Helicobacter pylori* (untreated); increase in non-specific diarrhoea when water quality exceeds 10^4 thermotolerant coliforms/100 ml	Evidence of parasitic protozoa found on wastewater-irrigated vegetable surfaces, but no direct evidence of disease transmission
Farm workers and their families	Significant risk of *Ascaris* infection for both adults and children in contact with untreated wastewater; risk remains, especially for children, when wastewater treated to <1 nematode egg per litre; increased risk of hookworm infection in workers	Increased risk of diarrhoeal disease in young children with wastewater contact if water quality exceeds 10^4 thermotolerant coliforms/100 ml; elevated risk of *Salmonella* infection in children exposed to untreated wastewater; elevated seroresponse to norovirus in adults exposed to partially treated wastewater	Risk of *Giardia intestinalis* infection was found insignificant for contact with both untreated and treated wastewater; increased risk of amoebiasis observed with contact with untreated wastewater
Nearby communities	*Ascaris* transmission not studied for sprinkler irrigation, but same as above for flood or furrow irrigation with heavy contact	Sprinkler irrigation with poor water quality (10^6–10^8 TC/100 ml) and high aerosol exposure associated with increased rates of infection; use of partially treated water (10^4–10^5 thermotolerant coliforms/100 ml or less) in sprinkler irrigation not found to be associated with increased viral infection rates	No data on transmission of protozoan infections during sprinkler irrigation with wastewater

TC, total coliforms

wastewater use in agriculture. In places where wastewater is used without adequate treatment, the greatest health risks are usually associated with intestinal helminths.

Table 2 presents a summary of the quantitative microbial risk assessment (QMRA) evidence for transmission of rotavirus infection due to different exposures. The risks for rotavirus transmission were always estimated to be higher than the risks associated with *Campylobacter* or *Cryptosporidium* infections.

Table 2. Summary of QMRA results for rotavirus[a] infection risks for different exposures

Exposure scenario	Water quality[b] (*E. coli*/100 ml wastewater or 100 g soil)	Median infection risks per person per year	Notes
Unrestricted irrigation (crop consumers)			
Lettuce	10^3–10^4	10^{-3}	100 g eaten raw per person every 2 days
			10–15 ml wastewater remaining on crop
Onion	10^3–10^4	5×10^{-2}	100 g eaten raw per person per week for 5 months
			1–5 ml wastewater remaining on crop
Restricted irrigation (farmers or other heavily exposed populations)			
Highly mechanized	10^5	10^{-3}	100 days exposure per year
			1–10 mg soil consumed per exposure
Labour intensive	10^3–10^4	10^{-3}	150–300 days exposure per year
			10–100 mg soil consumed per exposure

[a] Risks estimated for *Campylobacter* and *Cryptosporidium* are lower.
[b] Non-disinfected effluents.

Less evidence is available for health risks from chemicals. The evidence that is available is based on quantitative risk assessment and indicates that the uptake of chemicals by plants is highly dependent on the types of chemicals and the physical and chemical properties of soils.

Health-based targets

Health-based targets define a level of health protection that is relevant to each hazard. A health-based target can be based on a standard metric of disease, such as a DALY (e.g. 10^{-6} DALYs), or it can be based on an appropriate health outcome, such as the prevention of the transmission of vector-borne diseases resulting from exposures to wastewater use in agricultural practices. To achieve a health-based target, health protection measures are developed. Usually a health-based target can be achieved through a combination of health protection measures targeted at different components of the system. Figure 1 illustrates different combinations of health protection measures that can be used to achieve the 10^{-6} DALYs health-based target for excreta-related diseases.

Table 3 describes health-based targets for agriculture. The health-based targets for rotavirus are based on QMRA indicating the $\log_{10}$ pathogen reduction required to achieve 10^{-6} DALY for different exposures. To develop health-based targets for helminth infections, epidemiological evidence was used. This evidence demonstrated that excess helminth infections (for both product consumers and farmers) could not be measured when wastewater quality of ≤1 helminth egg per litre was used for irrigation. This level of health protection could also be met by treatment of wastewater or by a combination of wastewater treatment and washing of produce to protect consumers of raw vegetables; or by wastewater treatment and the use of personal protective equipment (shoes, gloves) to protect workers. When children less than 15 years old are exposed in the fields, either additional wastewater treatment (to achieve a wastewater quality of ≤0.1 helminth egg per litre) or the addition of other health protection measures (e.g. anthelminthic treatment) should be considered.

Table 3. Health-based targets for wastewater use in agriculture

Exposure scenario	Health-based target (DALY per person per year)	Log_{10} pathogen reduction needed[a]	Number of helminth eggs per litre
Unrestricted irrigation	$\leq 10^{-6}$ [a]		
Lettuce		6	≤ 1 [b,c]
Onion		7	≤ 1 [b,c]
Restricted irrigation	$\leq 10^{-6}$ [a]		
Highly mechanized		3	≤ 1 [b,c]
Labour intensive		4	≤ 1 [b,c]
Localized (drip) irrigation	$\leq 10^{-6}$ [a]		
High-growing crops		2	No recommendation[d]
Low-growing crops		4	≤ 1 [c]

[a] Rotavirus reduction. The health-based target can be achieved, for unrestricted and localized irrigation, by a 6–7 log unit pathogen reduction (obtained by a combination of wastewater treatment and other health protection measures); for restricted irrigation, it is achieved by a 2–3 log unit pathogen reduction.

[b] When children under 15 are exposed, additional health protection measures should be used (e.g. treatment to ≤ 0.1 egg per litre, protective equipment such as gloves or shoes/boots or chemotherapy).

[c] An arithmetic mean should be determined throughout the irrigation season. The mean value of ≤ 1 egg per litre should be obtained for at least 90% of samples in order to allow for the occasional high-value sample (i.e. with >10 eggs per litre). With some wastewater treatment processes (e.g. waste stabilization ponds), the hydraulic retention time can be used as a surrogate to assure compliance with ≤ 1 egg per litre.

[d] No crops to be picked up from the soil.

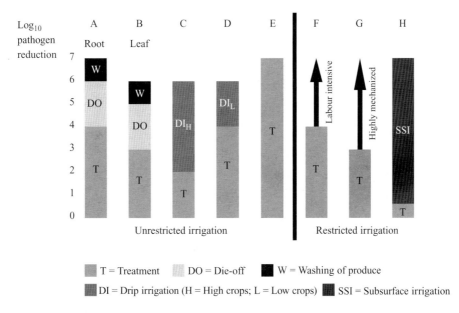

Figure 1
Examples of options for the reduction of viral, bacterial and protozoan pathogens by different combinations of health protection measures that achieve the health-based target of $\leq 10^{-6}$ DALYs per person per year

Table 4. Maximum tolerable soil concentrations of various toxic chemicals based on human health protection

Chemical	Soil concentration (mg/kg)
Element	
Antimony	36
Arsenic	8
Barium[a]	302
Beryllium[a]	0.2
Boron[a]	1.7
Cadmium	4
Fluorine	635
Lead	84
Mercury	7
Molybdenum[a]	0.6
Nickel	107
Selenium	6
Silver	3
Thallium[a]	0.3
Vanadium[a]	47
Organic compound	
Aldrin	0.48
Benzene	0.14
Chlordane	3
Chlorobenzene	211
Chloroform	0.47
2,4-D	0.25
DDT	1.54
Dichlorobenzene	15
Dieldrin	0.17
Dioxins	0.000 12
Heptachlor	0.18
Hexachlorobenzene	1.40
Lindane	12
Methoxychlor	4.27
PCBs	0.89
PAHs (as benzo[a]pyrene)	16
Pentachlorophenol	14
Phthalate	13 733
Pyrene	41
Styrene	0.68
2,4,5-T	3.82
Tetrachloroethane	1.25
Tetrachloroethylene	0.54
Toluene	12
Toxaphene	0.0013
Trichloroethane	0.68

[a] The computed numerical limits for these elements are within the ranges that are typical for soils.

Table 4 presents maximum soil concentrations for different chemicals based on health risk assessment. Concentrations of chemicals that impact agricultural productivity are described in Annex 1.

Health protection measures

A variety of health protection measures can be used to reduce health risks to consumers, workers and their families and local communities.

Hazards associated with the consumption of wastewater-irrigated products include excreta-related pathogens and some toxic chemicals. The risk from infectious pathogens is significantly reduced if foods are eaten after thorough cooking. Cooking has little or no impact on the concentrations of toxic chemicals that might be present. The following health protection measures have an impact on product consumers:

- wastewater treatment;
- crop restriction;
- waste application techniques that minimize contamination (e.g. drip irrigation);
- withholding periods to allow pathogen die-off after the last wastewater application;
- hygienic practices at food markets and during food preparation;
- health and hygiene promotion;
- produce washing, disinfection and cooking;
- chemotherapy and immunization.

Wastewater use activities may lead to the exposure of workers and their families to excreta-related diseases (including schistosomiasis), skin irritants and vector-borne diseases (in certain locations). Wastewater treatment is a control measure for excreta-related diseases, skin irritants and schistosomiasis but may not have much impact on vector-borne diseases. Other health protection measures for workers and their families include:

- use of personal protective equipment;
- access to safe drinking-water and sanitation facilities at farms;
- health and hygiene promotion;
- chemotherapy and immunization;
- disease vector and intermediate host control;
- reduced vector contact.

Local communities are at risk from the same hazards as workers, especially if they have access to wastewater-irrigated fields. If they do not have access to safe drinking-water, they may use contaminated irrigation water for drinking or for domestic purposes. Children may also play or swim in the contaminated water. Similarly, if wastewater irrigation activities result in increased vector breeding, then local communities may be affected by vector-borne diseases, even if they do not have direct access to the irrigated fields. To reduce health hazards, the following health protection measures for local communities may be used:

- wastewater treatment;
- restricted access to irrigated fields and hydraulic structures;
- access to safe recreational water, especially for adolescents;
- access to safe drinking-water and sanitation facilities in local communities;
- health and hygiene promotion;

- chemotherapy and immunization;
- disease vector and intermediate host control;
- reduced vector contact.

Monitoring and system assessment

Monitoring has three different purposes: validation, or proving that the system is capable of meeting its design requirements; operational monitoring, which provides information regarding the functioning of individual components of the health protection measures; and verification, which usually takes place at the end of the process to ensure that the system is achieving the specified targets.

The three functions of monitoring are each used for different purposes at different times. Validation is performed at the beginning when a new system is developed or when new processes are added and is used to test or prove that the system is capable of meeting the specified targets. Operational monitoring is used on a routine basis to indicate that processes are working as expected. Monitoring of this type relies on simple measurements that can be read quickly so that decisions can be made in time to remedy a problem. Verification is used to show that the end product (e.g. treated wastewater; crops) meets treatment targets (e.g. microbial quality specifications) and ultimately the health-based targets. Information from verification monitoring is collected periodically and thus would arrive too late to allow managers to make decisions to prevent a hazard break-through. However, verification monitoring can indicate trends over time (e.g. if the efficiency of a specific process was improving or decreasing).

The most effective means of consistently ensuring safety in the agricultural application of wastewater is through the use of a comprehensive risk assessment and risk management approach that encompasses all steps in the process from waste generation to treatment and use of wastewater to product use or consumption. This approach is captured in the Stockholm Framework. Three components of this approach are important for achieving the health-based targets: system assessment, identifying control measures and methods for monitoring them and developing a management plan.

Sociocultural aspects

Human behavioural patterns are a key determining factor in the transmission of excreta-related diseases. The social feasibility of changing certain behavioural patterns in order to introduce wastewater use schemes or to reduce disease transmission in existing schemes needs to be assessed on an individual project basis. Cultural beliefs vary so widely in different parts of the world that it is not possible to assume that any of the practices that have evolved in relation to wastewater use can be readily transferred elsewhere.

Closely associated with cultural beliefs is the public perception of wastewater use. Even when projects are technically well planned and all of the relevant health protection measures have been included, the project can fail if it does not account adequately for public perception.

Environmental aspects

Wastewater is an important source of water and nutrients for many farmers in arid and semi-arid climates. Sometimes it is the only water source available for agriculture. When wastewater use is well managed, it helps to recycle nutrients and water and therefore diminishes the cost of fertilizers or simply makes them accessible to farmers. Where wastewater treatment services are not provided, the use of wastewater in agriculture actually acts as a low-cost treatment method, taking advantage of the soil's capacity to naturally remove contamination. Therefore, the use of wastewater in irrigation helps to reduce downstream health and environmental impacts that would otherwise result if the wastewater were discharged directly into surface water bodies.

Nevertheless, wastewater use poses environmental risks. Possible effects and their relevance depend on each specific situation and how the wastewater is used. In many places, wastewater irrigation has arisen spontaneously and without planning — often the wastewater is untreated. In other situations, the use of wastewater in agriculture is strictly controlled. These practices will lead to different environmental impacts.

The properties of domestic wastewater and industrial wastewater differ. Generally, the use of domestic wastewater for irrigation poses less risk to the environment than the use of industrial wastewater, especially where industries use or produce highly toxic chemicals. Industrial discharges containing toxic chemicals are mixed with domestic wastewater in many countries, creating serious environmental problems and, where the wastewater is used for crop irrigation, endangering the health of the farmers and product consumers. Efforts should be made to reduce or eliminate practices that entail the mixing of domestic and industrial wastewater, particularly where wastewater is used for agriculture.

The use of wastewater in agriculture has the potential for both positive and negative environmental impacts. With careful planning and management, the use of wastewater in agriculture can be beneficial to the environment. Many of the environmental impacts (e.g. salinization of soil, contamination of water resources) can be reduced by good agricultural practices (as described in Annex 1).

Economic and financial considerations

Economic factors are especially important when the viability of a new scheme for the use of wastewater is being appraised, but even an economically worthwhile project can fail without careful financial planning.

Economic analysis and financial considerations are crucial for encouraging the safe use of wastewater. Economic analysis seeks to establish the economic feasibility of a project and enables comparisons between different options. The cost transfers to other sectors (e.g. the health and environmental impacts on downstream communities) also need to be included in a cost analysis. This can be facilitated by the use of multiple objective decision-making processes.

Financial planning looks at how the project is to be paid for. In establishing the financial feasibility of a project, it is important to determine the sources of revenues and clarify who will pay for what. The possibility to profitably sell products grown with wastewater or to sell the treated wastewater also needs analysis.

Policy aspects

The safe management of wastewater in agriculture is facilitated by appropriate policies, legislation, institutional frameworks and regulations at the international, national and local levels. In many countries where wastewater use in agriculture takes place, these frameworks are lacking.

Policy is the set of procedures, rules and allocation mechanisms that provide the basis for programmes and services. Policies set priorities, and associated strategies allocate resources for their implementation. Policies are implemented through four types of instruments: laws and regulations, economic measures, information and education programmes and assignments of rights and responsibilities for providing services.

In developing a national policy framework to facilitate safe wastewater use in agriculture, it is important to define the objectives of the policy, assess the current policy environment and develop a national approach. National approaches for safe wastewater use practices based on the WHO Guidelines will protect public health the most when they are integrated into comprehensive public health programmes that include other sanitary measures, such as health and hygiene promotion and improving access to safe drinking-water and adequate sanitation. Other complementary programmes, such as chemotherapy campaigns, should be accompanied by health promotion/education to change behaviours that would otherwise lead to reinfection (e.g. with intestinal helminths and other pathogens).

National approaches need to be adapted to the local sociocultural, environmental and economic circumstances, but they should be aimed at progressive improvement of public health. Interventions that address the greatest local health threats first should be given the highest priority. As resources and new data become available, additional health protection measures can be introduced.

The use of wastewater in agriculture can have one or more of several objectives. Defining these objectives is important for developing a national policy framework. The right policies can facilitate the safe use of wastewater in agriculture. Current policies often already exist that impact these activities, both negatively and positively. Conducting an assessment of current policies is often helpful for developing a new national policy or for revising existing policies. The assessment should take place at two levels: from the perspective of both a policy-maker and a project manager. Policy-makers will want to assess the national policies, legislation, institutional framework and regulations to ensure that they meet the national wastewater use objectives (e.g. maximize economic returns without endangering public health or the environment). Project coordinators will want to ensure that current and future waste use activities will be able to comply with all relevant national and local laws and regulations.

The main considerations are:

- *Policy:* Are there clear policies on the use of wastewater? Is wastewater use encouraged or discouraged?
- *Legislation:* Is the use of wastewater governed in legislation? What are the rights and responsibilities of different stakeholders? Does a defined jurisdiction exist on the use of wastewater?
- *Institutional framework:* Which ministry/agency, organizations, etc. have the authority to control the use of wastewater at the national level and at the district/community level? Are the responsibilities of different ministries/agencies clear? Is there one lead ministry, or are there multiple ministries/agencies with overlapping jurisdictions? Which ministry/agency is responsible for developing regulations? Which ministry/agency monitors compliance with regulations? Which ministry/agency enforces the regulations?
- *Regulations:* Do regulations exist? Are the current regulations adequate to meet wastewater use objectives (protect public health, prevent environmental damage, meet produce quality standards for domestic and international trade, preserve livelihoods, conserve water and nutrients, etc.)? Are the current regulations being implemented? Is regulatory compliance being enforced?

It is easier to make regulations than to enforce them. In drafting new regulations (or in choosing which existing ones to enforce), it is important to plan for the institutions, staff and resources necessary to ensure that the regulations are followed. It is important to ensure that the regulations are realistic and achievable in the context in which they are to be applied. It will often be advantageous to adopt a gradual approach or to test a new set of regulations by persuading a local administration to pass them as by-laws before they are extended to the rest of the country.

Planning and implementation

Planning and implementation of wastewater irrigation programmes require a comprehensive progressive approach that responds to the greatest health priorities first. Strategies for developing national programmes should include elements on communication to stakeholders, interaction with stakeholders and the collection and use of data.

Additionally, planning for projects at a local level requires an assessment of several important underlying factors. The sustainability of wastewater use in agriculture relies on the assessment and understanding of eight important criteria: health, economic feasibility, social impact and public perception, financial feasibility, environmental impact, market feasibility, institutional feasibility and technical feasibility.

1
INTRODUCTION

This volume of the *Guidelines for the safe use of wastewater, excreta and greywater* describes the present state of knowledge regarding possible health impacts of wastewater use in agriculture. This chapter describes the objectives and general considerations related to the Guidelines and their target audience. It also provides some definitions and presents an overview of what World Health Organization (WHO) water-related guidelines are and how they relate to wastewater use in agriculture. Driving forces that impact wastewater use in agriculture are also described.

1.1 Objectives and general considerations

The primary objective of these Guidelines is to maximize the public health benefits of wastewater use in agriculture. To achieve this objective, strategies are needed, in the context of wastewater use, to minimize the transmission of infectious agents and the exposure to toxic chemicals for farmers and their families, for local communities and for product consumers. This can be achieved by minimizing human exposure to pathogens and toxic chemicals in the wastewater. Other objectives include, for example, managing the use of wastewater to maximize crop production and minimize environmental impacts. For these aspects, the reader is referred to publications by the Food and Agriculture Organization of the United Nations (FAO) (e.g. Ayers & Westcot, 1985; Pescod, 1992; Ongley, 1996; Westcot, 1997a, 1997b; Allen et al., 1998; Tanji & Kielen, 2002; see also Annex 1) and the United Nations Environment Programme's Global Programme of Action for the Protection of the Marine Environment from Land-based Activities (http://www.gpa.unep.org/).

The Guidelines are based on the development and use of health-based targets. Health-based targets establish a goal of attaining a certain level of health protection in an exposed population. This level of health can then be achieved by using a combination of management approaches (e.g. crop restriction, application techniques, human exposure control) and water quality targets to arrive at the specified health outcome. Achieving the health-based targets requires monitoring and system assessment, defining institutional and supervisory responsibilities, system documentation and independent confirmation that the system is working. Thus, the guidelines consist of both good practice advice and water quality specifications and may include:

- a level of management;
- a concentration of a constituent that does not represent a significant risk to the health of members of important user groups;
- a condition under which such transmissions or exposures are unlikely to occur; or
- a combination of the last two.

The Guidelines provide an integrated preventive management framework (see Box 1.1 and discussion on the Stockholm Framework in chapter 2) for safety applied from the point of waste generation to consumption of products grown with the wastewater. They describe reasonable minimum requirements of good practice to protect the health of the people using wastewater or consuming products grown with it, and they derive health-based targets and explain their adaptation. Neither the minimum good practices nor the health-based targets are mandatory limits. In order to define such limits, it is necessary to consider the Guidelines in the context of national environmental, social, economic and cultural conditions (WHO, 2004a).

Box 1.1 What are the Guidelines?

The WHO Guidelines are an integrated preventive management framework for maximizing the public health benefits of wastewater use in agriculture. The Guidelines are built around a health component and an implementation component. Health protection is dependent on both elements.

Health component:
- defines a level of health protection that is expressed as a health-based target for each hazard;
- identifies health protection measures that, used collectively, can achieve the specified health-based target.

Implementation component:
- establishes monitoring and system assessment procedures;
- defines institutional and supervisory responsibilities;
- requires system documentation;
- requires confirmation by independent surveillance.

The approach followed in these Guidelines is intended to support the establishment of national standards and regulations that can be readily implemented and enforced and are protective of public health. Each country should review its needs and capacities in developing a regulatory framework. Successful implementation of the Guidelines will require a broad-based policy framework that includes positive and negative incentives to alter behaviour and monitor and improve situations. Intersectoral coordination and cooperation at national and local levels and the development of suitable skills and expertise will facilitate implementation of the Guidelines.

In many situations, it will not be possible to fully implement the Guidelines at once. The Guidelines set target values designed in such a way as to allow progressive implementation. They are to be achieved over time in an orderly manner, depending on the current reality and the existing resources of each individual country or region. The greatest threats to health should be given the highest priority and addressed first. Over time, it should be possible to adjust risk management strategies to strive for the continual improvement of public health.

Ultimately, the judgement of safety — or what is a tolerable level of risk in particular circumstances — is a matter in which society as a whole has a role to play. The final judgement as to whether the benefit from using any of the guidelines and health-based targets as national or local standards justifies the cost is for each country to decide, in the context of national public health, environmental and socioeconomic realities and international trade regulations.

1.2 Target audience, definitions and scope

The revised *Guidelines for the safe use of wastewater, excreta and greywater* will be useful to all those concerned with issues relating to the safe use of wastewater, excreta and greywater, public health and water and waste management. The target audience may include environmental and public health scientists, educators, researchers, engineers, policy-makers and those responsible for developing standards and regulations.

This volume of the Guidelines addresses the use of wastewater in agriculture. These Guidelines focus on wastewater consisting of domestic sewage that does not contain industrial effluents at levels that could pose threats to the functioning of the sewerage system, treatment plant, public health or the environment. The ability to use wastewater with significant concentrations of industrial chemicals in agriculture should be determined on a case-by-case basis. Sludge derived from the treatment of municipal or industrial wastewater is not included in the scope of this document. Definitions of common terms used in this volume are presented in the glossary in Annex 4.

The public health aspects and the health-based targets for wastewater-irrigated agriculture are applicable to cases where wastewater is used indirectly (i.e. discharged into surface water, which is then abstracted and used for agriculture). In many areas, surface waters such as rivers used for irrigation may be highly contaminated, with properties similar to those of diluted wastewater.

1.3 Driving forces behind increasing wastewater use

Wastewater is being increasingly used for the irrigation of agricultural crops in both developing and industrialized countries. The principal forces driving the increasing use of wastewater are:

- increasing water scarcity and stress, and degradation of freshwater resources resulting from improper disposal of wastewater;
- population increase and related increased demand for food and fibre;
- a growing recognition of the resource value of wastewater and the nutrients it contains;
- the Millennium Development Goals (MDGs), especially the goals for ensuring environmental sustainability and eliminating poverty and hunger.

1.3.1 Increasing water scarcity and stress

Fresh water is already scarce in many parts of the world, and population growth in water-scarce regions will further increase its value. In 1995, 31 countries were classified as water-scarce or water-stressed, and it is estimated that 48 and 54 countries will fall into these categories by 2025 and 2050, respectively. These numbers do not include people living in arid regions of large countries where there is enough water but it is poorly distributed — e.g. China, India and the United States of America (China is predicted to reach water scarcity by 2050 and India by 2025) (Hinrichsen, Robey & Upadhyay, 1998). Growing competition between agriculture and urban areas for high-quality freshwater supplies, particularly in arid, semi-arid and densely populated regions, will increase the pressure on this resource.

1.3.2 Increasing population

Within the next 50 years, it is estimated that more than 40% of the world's population will live in countries facing water stress or water scarcity (Figure 1.1). Most population growth is expected to occur in urban and periurban areas in developing countries (United Nations Population Division, 2002). For example, most of the 19 cities predicted to grow the most rapidly during 2000–2015 (with populations expected to more than double in this period) are in chronically water-short regions of developing countries (United Nations Population Division, 2002).

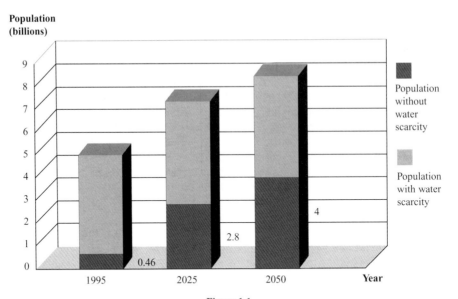

Figure 1.1
Population living in water-scarce and water-stressed countries, 1995–2050
(Hinrichsen, Robey & Upadhyay, 1998; United Nations Population Division, 2000)

As populations grow and become more urban, water use and consequent wastewater generation increase. For example, water usage in North America increased by approximately 800% during 1900–1995, and global water use in 2000 was estimated to be nearly three times what it was in 1950 (Shiklomanov, 1998). Annual household water consumption ranges from approximately 1 m^3 per person in the rural tropics without piped water supplies to >200 m^3 per person in urban areas in the United States of America (Gleick, 2000).

The growth of urban populations, especially in developing countries, will influence the production, treatment and use of wastewater in several ways:

- Higher population densities in urban and periurban areas will generate more waste (much of which will be discharged into the environment with little or no treatment).
- Urban populations consume more water than rural populations, which also increases the amount of wastewater produced.
- Sewerage systems become dominant in urban areas, because on-site waste disposal is not always feasible in many densely populated areas.
- Urban agriculture (with wastewater as a common water source) will play a more important role in supplying food to cities.
- Municipal wastewater will become the sole water source for many farmers in water-stressed areas close to cities.

1.3.3 Wastewater as a resource

Agriculture is the single largest user of fresh water in the world, accounting for nearly 70% (>90% in some countries) of all extractions of fresh water worldwide (Gleick, 2000; FAO, 2002). As fresh water becomes increasingly scarce due to population growth, urbanization and climate change, the use of wastewater in agriculture will increase even more.

At least 10% of the world's population is thought to consume foods produced by irrigation with wastewater (Smit & Nasr, 1992). The water and nutrient value of wastewater are important resources for farmers in both industrialized and developing countries. For example, in California, USA, approximately 67% of wastewater is reclaimed and used for crop or landscape irrigation (California State Water Resources Control Board, 2003), and in Israel the figure is approximately 75% (Arlosoroff, 2002). Wastewater is approximately 99% water. Where households are connected to piped water supplies, wastewater is generated at a rate of 35–200 litres per person per day (12–70 m^3 per person per year), depending on the water supply service level, climate and water availability (Helmer & Hespanhol, 1997). In a semi-arid area, a city of one million people would produce enough wastewater to irrigate approximately 1500–3500 ha.

The use of wastewater for crop irrigation reduces the use of artificial fertilizers and is thus an important form of nutrient recycling. At an irrigation rate of 1.5 m/year (i.e 1.5 m^3 of irrigation water per m^2 of field area per year), a typical requirement in a semi-arid climate, treated municipal wastewater can supply 225 kg of nitrogen and 45 kg of phosphorus per hectare per year. Thus, supplementary fertilization needs can be reduced (or even eliminated) for some crops, with a consequent increase in farmers' income. Additionally, using the nutrients available in wastewater reduces the environmental impacts associated with the mining (phosphorus) and production of artificial fertilizers.

1.3.4 The Millennium Development Goals

The United Nations General Assembly adopted the MDGs on 8 September 2000 (United Nations General Assembly, 2000). The MDGs most relevant to the agricultural use of wastewater are Goals 1 and 7.

Goal 1: Eliminate extreme poverty and hunger

Wastewater irrigation can contribute to the achievement of this MDG, as more food crops can be produced, allowing farmers' incomes to rise. Irrigation with wastewater is potentially very profitable for farmers. For example, in some areas in Pakistan, farmers willingly pay higher fees (US$ 350–940 per year) for access to wastewater compared with access to fresh water (US$ 170 per year), since it allows them to harvest three crops per year instead of one. Despite the higher fees, farmers with access to wastewater earn US$ 300 more per year than farmers using fresh water (Ensink, Simmons & van der Hoek, 2004). In the Guanajuato River basin in Mexico, 140 ha of land are irrigated with wastewater, which provides local farmers with nutrients estimated to be worth US$ 135 per hectare per year. For poor farmers, this is a substantial amount of money, which would otherwise have been used to purchase chemical fertilizers or resulted in lower yields (Future Harvest, 2001).

Irrigation with wastewater produces higher crop yields than irrigation with fresh water, even when artificial fertilizers are used. For example, in Nagpur, India, irrigation with waste stabilization pond effluents yielded 28, 8, 47, 30 and 42% more wheat, moong beans (type of lentils), rice, potato and cotton, respectively, than irrigation with fresh water supplemented with fertilizer containing nitrogen, phosphorus and potassium (Shende et al., 1985). In Dakar, Senegal, farmers who used only wastewater for irrigation had higher yields for most vegetable crops than farmers who used piped water and chemical fertilizers. Moreover, using wastewater resulted in a shorter crop production time for some crops (e.g. lettuce), and thus farmers who used wastewater could produce nine lettuce crops per year compared with six for farmers who used groundwater (Faruqui, Niang & Redwood, 2004).

Higher yields of food crops mean improved food availability. The economics of supply and demand indicate that the more food there is, the lower its price; thus, more people (especially poor people) can buy more food and be at least less hungry. Currently, poor households spend a larger proportion (50–80%) of their income on food and water compared with non-poor households (Lipton, 1983; World Food Programme, 1995). For example, based on household surveys in India, Buechler & Devi (2003) found that per capita expenditure on food averaged 30, 44 and 66% in urban, periurban and rural areas, respectively. Without access to resources such as wastewater, many poor families would not be able to meet their nutritional needs or would have to spend more money on food and less on other health-promoting activities, such as primary health care or education. It is therefore important to use a risk–benefit approach when developing guidelines for wastewater and excreta use in agriculture. This approach is followed in chapter 4 of these Guidelines.

Goal 7: Ensure environmental sustainability
Wastewater irrigation contributes to environmental sustainability by using the nutrients and water in wastewaters beneficially for increased crop production. Consequently, the quantity of untreated wastewater discharged into the aquatic environment will be reduced. It would otherwise lead to the degradation of water quality and act as a vehicle for disease transmission to users of polluted waters. The recognition of wastewater as an integral and reliable component of a nation's water resources (see section 1.3.3) and its equitable distribution as a preferred water for irrigation are essential for the efficient allocation and use of freshwater resources, especially in water-short and water-scarce areas.

Wastewater can also be used to protect groundwater for irrigation uses. When the water in coastal aquifers is pumped out at excessive rates, salt water from the ocean or sea flows into the aquifer, replacing the extracted fresh water. Treated wastewater can act as a barrier to saline intrusion when it is pumped into the aquifer, thus preventing the water from becoming brackish and preserving its value for food production. Aquifer recharge with treated wastewater is becoming more common in many coastal areas where aquifers are depleted through overextraction (Mills et al., 1998; National Research Council, 1998).

1.4 Organization of this Guidelines document

The structure of this volume is illustrated in Figure 1.2. Chapter 2 provides an overview of the Stockholm Framework. Chapter 3 provides the epidemiological, microbial and risk assessment bases for the Guidelines, which are formally developed in chapter 4 as health-based targets. Chapter 5 reviews the health protection measures that can be used to achieve the health-based targets. Chapter 6 reviews monitoring requirements. Chapter 7 presents the sociocultural and public perception aspects that need to be considered in wastewater use in agriculture. Chapter 8 describes environmental aspects of wastewater use in agriculture. Chapter 9 presents information on economic and financial aspects that need to be considered. Chapter 10 discusses policy aspects, and Chapter 11 reviews planning and implementation issues. Annex 1 briefly discusses good agricultural practice in relation to wastewater irrigation, and Annex 2 presents a summary of studies concerning the impact of heavy metals on the environment associated with wastewater irrigation. Health impact assessment with regard to wastewater use in agriculture is discussed in Annex 3.

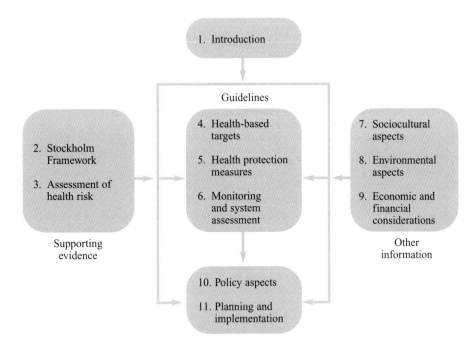

Figure 1.2
Structure of Volume 2 of the *Guidelines for the safe use of wastewater, excreta and greywater*

Annex 4 is a glossary of terms used in the *Guidelines for the safe use of wastewater, excreta and greywater.*

The Stockholm Framework is an integrated approach that combines risk assessment and risk management to control water-related diseases. Although it was developed for infectious diseases, it can be applied to illnesses resulting from water-related exposures to toxic chemicals. This chapter contains a summary of the components of the Framework and how it applies to assessing and managing risks associated with the use of wastewater in agriculture. Specific components of the Framework are discussed in more detail in other chapters.

2.1 A harmonized approach to risk assessment/management

Following an expert meeting in Stockholm, Sweden, WHO published *Water quality: Guidelines, standards and health — Assessment of risk and risk management for water-related infectious disease* (Fewtrell & Bartram, 2001). This report provides a harmonized framework for the development of health-based guidelines and standards for water- and sanitation-related microbial hazards. The Stockholm Framework involves the assessment of health risks prior to the setting of health-based targets and the development of guideline values, defining basic control approaches and evaluating the impact of these combined approaches on public health (Figure 2.1; Table 2.1).

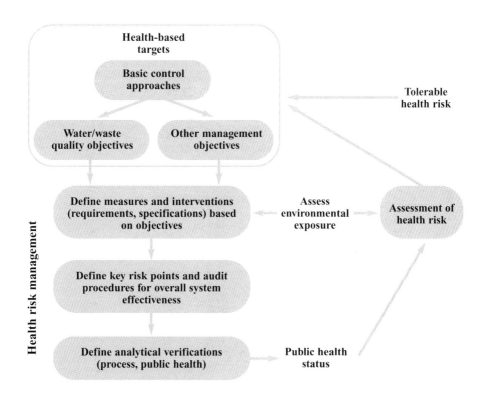

Figure 2.1
The Stockholm Framework for developing harmonized guidelines for the management of water-related infectious disease (adapted from Bartram, Fewtrell & Stenström, 2001)

Table 2.1 Elements and important considerations of the Stockholm Framework

Framework component	Process	Considerations
Assessment of health risk	Epidemiological studies	Best estimate of risk — not overly conservative
	QMRA	Health outcomes presented in DALYs facilitates comparison of risks across different exposures and priority setting
		Assessment of risk is an iterative process — risk should be periodically reassessed based on new data or changing conditions
		Risk assessment (QMRA) is a tool for estimating risk and should be supported by other data (e.g. outbreak investigations, epidemiological evidence and studies of environmental behaviour of microbes)
		Process dependent on quality of data
		Risk assessment needs to account for short-term underperformance
Tolerable health risk/health-based targets	Health-based target setting linked to risk assessment	Needs to be realistic and achievable within the constraints of each setting
		Set based on a risk–benefit approach; should consider cost-effectiveness of different available interventions
		Should take sensitive subpopulations into account
		Reference pathogens should be selected for relevance to contamination, control challenges and health significance (it may be necessary to select more than one reference pathogen)
		Health-based targets establish a desired health outcome
Health risk management	Define water/waste quality objectives	Health-based targets should be the basis for selecting risk management strategies; exposure prevention occurs through a combination of good practices (e.g. wastewater treatment, use of personal protective equipment, etc.) and appropriate water quality objectives (e.g. *Escherichia coli* and helminth eggs; see chapter 4)
	Define other management objectives	
	Define measures and interventions	
	Define key risk points and audit procedures	Risk points should be defined and used to anticipate and minimize health risks; parameters for monitoring can be set up around risk points
	Define analytical verifications	A multiple-barrier approach should be used
		Risk management strategies need to address rare or catastrophic events
		Validation of the effectiveness of the health protection measures is needed to ensure that the system is capable of meeting the health-based targets; validation is needed when a new system is developed or additional barriers/technologies are added
		Monitoring — overall emphasis should be given to periodic inspection/auditing and to simple measurements that can be rapidly and frequently made to inform management
		Analytical verifications may include testing wastewater and/or plants for *E. coli* or helminth eggs to confirm that the treatment processes are working to the desired level
		Verification data can be used to make necessary adjustments to the risk management process to improve safety

Table 2.1 (continued)

Framework component	Process	Considerations
Public health status	Public health surveillance	Need to evaluate effectiveness of risk management interventions on specific health outcomes (through both investigation of disease outbreaks and evaluation of background disease levels)
		Public health outcome monitoring provides the information needed to fine-tune the risk management process through an iterative process; procedures for estimating the burden of disease will facilitate monitoring health outcomes due to specific exposures
		Burden of disease estimates can be used to place water-related exposures in the wider public health context to enable prioritization of risk management decisions

Source: Adapted from Carr & Bartram (2004).

The Framework encourages countries to take into consideration their local social, cultural, economic and environmental circumstances and compare the wastewater- and excreta-associated health risks with risks that may result from microbial exposures through other water and sanitation routes and additional exposures (e.g. through food, hygienic practices, etc.). This approach facilitates the management of infectious diseases in an integrated, holistic fashion and not in isolation from other diseases or exposure routes. Disease outcomes from different exposure routes can be compared by using a common metric, such as disability adjusted life years (DALYs), or normalized for a population over a time period (see Box 2.1).

Box 2.1 Disability adjusted life years (DALYs)

DALYs are a measure of the health of a population or burden of disease due to a specific disease or risk factor. DALYs attempt to measure the time lost because of disability or death from a disease compared with a long life free of disability in the absence of the disease. DALYs are calculated by adding the years of life lost to premature death to the years lived with a disability. Years of life lost are calculated from age-specific mortality rates and the standard life expectancies of a given population. Years lived with a disability are calculated from the number of cases multiplied by the average duration of the disease and a severity factor ranging from 1 (death) to 0 (perfect health) based on the disease (e.g. watery diarrhoea has a severity factor ranging from 0.09 to 0.12, depending on the age group) (Murray & Lopez, 1996; Prüss & Havelaar, 2001). DALYs are an important tool for comparing health outcomes, because they account not only for acute health effects but also for delayed and chronic effects — including morbidity and mortality (Bartram, Fewtrell & Stenström, 2001).

When risk is described in DALYs, different health outcomes (e.g. cancer vs giardiasis) can be compared and risk management decisions can be prioritized.

WHO water- and sanitation-related guidelines have been developed in accordance with the principles of the Stockholm Framework. The third edition of the WHO *Guidelines for drinking-water quality* (WHO, 2004a) and volumes 1 and 2 of the WHO *Guidelines for safe recreational water environments* (WHO, 2003a, 2005) have both incorporated its harmonized approach to risk assessment and management. The following sections describe the individual elements of the Stockholm Framework, as illustrated in Figure 2.1, and how they specifically relate to the use of wastewater.

Some of the elements related to wastewater use in agriculture are discussed in more detail in subsequent chapters of this document.

2.2 Assessment of environmental exposure

The assessment of environmental exposure is an important input to both risk assessment and risk management. Environmental exposure assessment is a process that looks at the hazards in the environment and evaluates different transmission and exposure routes to human (or animal) populations. Table 2.2 describes the hazards associated with the use of wastewater in agriculture, the primary hazards being pathogens and certain chemicals. Treatment of wastewater to varying degrees can significantly reduce the concentrations of some contaminants (e.g. excreta-derived pathogens and some chemicals) (see chapter 5) and thus the risk of disease transmission. Other strategies are necessary to prevent the transmission of vector-borne diseases.

Table 2.2 Examples of hazards associated with wastewater use in agriculture

Hazard	Exposure route	Relative importance	Comments
Excreta-related pathogens			
Bacteria (*E. coli*, *Vibrio cholerae*, *Salmonella* spp., *Shigella* spp.)	Contact Consumption	Low–high	Can survive in the environment long enough to pose health risks. Contamination of crops has led to disease outbreaks.
			Produce washing/disinfection and cooking reduce the risk. Poor personal hygiene after wastewater contact will increase the risk of infection/disease.
Helminths			
- Soil-transmitted (*Ascaris*, hookworms, *Taenia* spp.)	Contact Consumption	Low–high	Present in areas where sanitation and hygiene standards are low. Risk depends on how wastewater is treated, if shoes are worn, if food is cooked before eating, etc. Eggs can survive for a very long time in the environment.
- Schistosomes (trematode bloodflukes)	Contact	Nil–high	Schistosomes are present only in certain geographic regions and require suitable intermediate hosts. Schistosomiasis is transmitted through contact with contaminated water in endemic areas.
Protozoa (*Giardia intestinalis*, *Cryptosporidium*, *Entamoeba* spp.)	Contact Consumption	Low– medium	Can survive in the environment long enough to pose health risks. Limited evidence of disease outbreaks.
			Produce washing/disinfection and cooking reduce the risk. Poor personal hygiene after wastewater contact will increase the risk of infection/disease.
Viruses (hepatitis A virus, hepatitis E virus, adenovirus, rotavirus, norovirus)	Contact Consumption	Low– high	Can survive in the environment long enough to pose health risks. Contamination of crops has led to disease outbreaks.

Table 2.2 (continued)

Hazard	Exposure route	Relative importance	Comments
Viruses (hepatitis A virus, hepatitis E virus, adenovirus, rotavirus, norovirus) *(continued)*			Produce washing/disinfection and cooking reduce the risk. Poor personal hygiene after wastewater contact will increase the risk of infection/disease. In areas with poor sanitation and hygiene standards, most people are infected as children and develop immunity. May pose more of a health risk for local people who are not exposed as children or for tourists without immunity to local diseases.
Skin irritants	Contact	Medium– high	Skin diseases such as contact dermatitis (eczema) have been reported after heavy contact with untreated wastewater. Cause has not yet been determined but is likely due to a mixture of microbial and chemical agents. May also be caused by cyanobacterial toxins in some situations.
Vector-borne pathogens (*Plasmodium* spp., dengue virus, *Wuchereria bancrofti*, Japanese encephalitis virus)	Vector contact	Nil–medium	Limited to geographic areas where the pathogen is endemic and suitable vectors are present. Risk is mainly associated with water resource development (i.e. development of reservoirs and irrigation systems) and usually not specifically with wastewater use in agriculture. Lymphatic filariasis is the exception, as its vectors breed in organically polluted water.
Chemicals			
Heavy metals (arsenic, cadmium, lead, mercury)	Consumption	Low	Heavy metals may accumulate in some plants, but rarely to levels considered unsafe.
Halogenated hydrocarbons (dioxins, furans, PCBs)	Consumption	Low	Concentration of these substances is generally low in wastewater (but may be higher in sludge). These substances are usually adsorbed by soil particles and not taken up by plants.
Pesticides (aldrin, DDT)	Contact Consumption	Low	Risk is related to agricultural practices. Wastewater generally does not contain high concentrations of these substances.

Sources: Blumenthal et al. (2000a, 2000b); WHO (2004q); van der Hoek et al. (2005).

Raw wastewater contains a variety of human pathogens (see chapter 3). The concentrations of pathogens vary from region to region and over time. Pathogen concentrations will be at the highest levels in areas where faecal–oral disease is widely endemic. If excreta-related disease outbreaks occur, then concentrations of the causative pathogen may also reach higher levels in the wastewater and excreta.

Many pathogens are capable of survival (and sometimes multiplication) in the environment (e.g. water, plants, soil) for periods long enough to allow transmission to humans. Several factors influence their die-off, including temperature, moisture, exposure to ultraviolet radiation, time, absence of appropriate intermediate hosts, type of plant, etc.

The primary pathways of transmission of or exposure to pathogens or contaminants associated with the use of wastewater in agriculture are:

- human contact with the wastewater (or contaminated crops) before, during or after irrigation (farmers, their families, vendors, local communities);
- inhalation of wastewater aerosols (workers, local communities);
- consumption of contaminated wastewater-irrigated products;
- consumption of drinking-water contaminated as a result of wastewater use activities (e.g. chemical or pathogen contamination of aquifers or surface waters);
- consumption of animals (e.g. beef or pork) or animal products (e.g. milk) that have been contaminated through exposure to wastewater;
- vector-borne disease transmission resulting from the development and management of wastewater irrigation schemes and waste stabilization ponds.

The concentrations of toxic chemicals will vary from place to place and will usually depend on the number and types of industries that discharge their wastes into the wastewater and the degree to which they treat their wastes prior to discharge.

2.3 Assessment of health risk

Assessing the risk associated with human exposure to pathogens in wastewater for agriculture can be carried out with information gained from epidemiological studies and quantitative microbial risk assessments (QMRA). As they can provide complementary information, ideally, risk assessment is carried out with both.

Epidemiological studies aim to assess the health risks associated with the use of wastewater by comparing the level of disease in the exposed population (which uses wastewater or consumes products grown with it) with that in an unexposed or control population. The difference in disease levels may then be attributed to the practice of using the wastewater, provided that the two populations compared are similar in all other respects, including socioeconomic status and ethnicity. Confounding factors and bias that may affect results need to be addressed in the study by careful selection of the study participants. Blumenthal & Peasey (2002) conducted a review of epidemiological studies concerning the use of wastewater in agriculture, the results of which are presented in chapter 3.

QMRA can be used to estimate the risk to human health by predicting infection or illness rates given densities of particular pathogens, measured or estimated rates of ingestion and appropriate dose–response models for the exposed population. QMRA provides a technique for estimating the risks from a specific pathogen associated with a specific exposure pathway. It is a sensitive tool that can estimate risks that would be difficult and costly to measure and therefore provides an important complement to epidemiological investigations, which are less sensitive and more difficult to perform. QMRA consists of four steps, which are outlined in Table 2.2. Examples of QMRAs used to estimate health risks for the use of wastewater under different scenarios are provided in chapter 3.

Table 2.2 Risk assessment paradigm for any human health effect[a]

Step	Aim
1. Hazard identification	To describe acute and chronic human health effects associated with any particular hazard, including pathogens or toxic chemicals
2. Hazard characterization	Dose–response assessment, to characterize the relationship between various doses administered and the incidence of the health effect, including underlying mechanisms and extrapolation from model systems to humans
3. Exposure assessment	To determine the size and nature of the population exposed and the route, amount and duration of the exposure
4. Risk characterization	To integrate the information from exposure, dose–response and hazard identification steps in order to estimate the magnitude of the public health problem and to evaluate variability and uncertainty

Source: Adapted from WHO (2003a).
[a] Can be used for both chemicals and microbial pathogens.

2.4 Tolerable health risk

The management of health risk is context-specific; there is no universally applicable risk management formula. In setting guidelines for the use of wastewater, logic dictates that the overall levels of health protection should be comparable with those for other water-related exposures (e.g. through drinking-water). Standards for drinking-water consider illnesses that might result from exposures to both chemicals and microbial pathogens. The comparison of different adverse health outcomes, such as cancer, diarrhoea, etc., is facilitated by the use of a common metric (i.e. DALYs; see Box 2.1 and chapter 4). Significant experience has now been gained in such comparisons (WHO, 2003a).

For carcinogenic chemicals in drinking-water, WHO guideline values have been set at a 10^{-5} upper-bound excess risk (WHO, 2004a). This means that there would be a maximum of one excess case of cancer per 100 000 of the population ingesting drinking-water that contained the chemical at the guideline concentration over a lifetime. The disease burden associated with this level of risk and adjusted for the severity of the illness is approximately 1×10^{-6} DALY (1 µDALY) per person per year (WHO, 2004a). This level of disease burden can be compared with a mild but more frequent illness, such as self-limiting diarrhoea caused by a microbial pathogen. The estimated disease burden associated with mild diarrhoea (e.g. with a case fatality rate of approximately 1×10^{-5}) at an annual disease risk of 1 in 1000 (10^{-3}) (1 in 10 lifetime risk) is also about 1×10^{-6} DALY (1 µDALY) per person per year (WHO, 2004a).

2.5 Health-based targets

Health-based targets should be part of overall public health policy, taking into account status and trends and the contribution of wastewater use to the transmission of infectious disease, both in individual settings and within overall health management. The purpose of setting targets is to mark milestones to guide and chart progress towards a predetermined health goal. To ensure effective health protection and improvement, targets need to be realistic and relevant to local conditions, including financial, technical and institutional resources. Such conditions include the nature and seriousness of local illness, population behaviour, exposure patterns and sociocultural, economic, environmental and technical aspects, as well as health risks from other diseases, including those that are not associated with wastewater use (WHO, 2003a). This normally implies periodic review and updating of priorities and targets and, in turn, that norms and standards should be revised to take account of these factors and the changes in available information (WHO, 2004a).

A health-based target uses the tolerable risk of disease as a baseline to set specific performance targets that will reduce the risk of disease to this level. Exposure to different concentrations of pathogens or toxic chemicals through wastewater contact or through consumption of wastewater-irrigated products is associated with a certain level of risk. Reducing this risk thus involves minimizing exposures to pathogens and chemicals.

Health-based targets can be specified in terms of combinations of different components or single parameters, including:

- *Health outcome:* as determined by epidemiological studies, public health surveillance or QMRA (DALYs or absence of a specific disease);
- *Wastewater quality:* such as concentrations of viable intestinal nematode eggs and/or *E. coli*;
- *Performance:* such as a performance target for removal of microbial or chemical contaminants (e.g. a percentage removal of pathogens through a combination of treatment requirements, water quality standards and wastewater application techniques; see chapters 4 and 5); performance may be assessed through validation (see chapter 6) or approximated by other parameters — retention time in ponds; turbidity; suspended solids, etc., for monitoring purposes;
- *Specified technology:* specified treatment process, etc., either in general or with reference to specific circumstances of use.

2.6 Risk management

Risk management strategies can be developed to ensure achievement of health-based targets. Pollution prevention, especially for chemicals, should also be considered in risk management strategies. Measures and interventions will be different based on the wastewater use objective. The most effective means of consistently ensuring safety in wastewater use in agriculture is through the use of a comprehensive risk assessment and risk management approach that encompasses all steps in the process, from the generation and use of wastewater to product consumption. This approach is captured in the Stockholm Framework. Three components of this approach are important for achieving the health-based targets: system assessment, identifying control measures and methods for monitoring them and developing a management plan (these procedures are discussed in more detail in chapter 6).

Performance targets to achieve exposure reductions for unrestricted versus restricted irrigation will vary. For example, it may be determined that a 99.99% reduction in exposure to pathogens is needed to achieve the health-based target for unrestricted irrigation, while a 99% reduction is needed to achieve the health-based target for restricted irrigation. The targets in the first case could be met by a combination of treatment plus localized irrigation and in the second case by just treatment (plus exposure prevention for workers and local communities) (see Figure 2.2). Chapters 4 and 5 present more information on exposure reductions that may be achieved by specific management approaches.

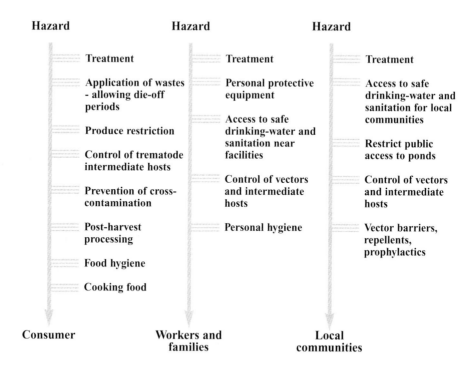

Figure 2.2
Examples of hazard barriers for wastewater use in agriculture

Figure 2.2 shows examples of risk management strategies for wastewater use in agriculture to prevent exposures to pathogens and toxic chemicals by constructing multiple barriers (additional strategies are discussed in chapter 5). They may include combinations of the following:

- *Wastewater treatment:* to remove pathogens and toxic chemicals to levels that do not exceed tolerable risks or that can be combined with other measures to achieve the health-based targets;
- *Produce restriction:* growing plants that either are not eaten directly by humans or are always processed (cooked) prior to consumption;
- *Application:* using wastewater/excreta application techniques that reduce exposures of workers and contamination of products, or allowing adequate periods between waste application and harvest to allow pathogen die-off (e.g. drip irrigation, withholding periods, buffer zones);
- *Exposure control methods:* limiting public access to irrigated fields, workers wearing protective clothing, good personal hygienic practices, such as hand-washing with soap to remove contaminants after contact with wastewater or products contaminated with them;
- *Produce washing/disinfection/cooking:* normal washing of produce in the houseold with safe drinking-water or using chemical disinfectants can reduce contamination and potential exposures to pathogens and some chemicals; cooking food thoroughly prior to consumption will inactivate most, if not all, pathogens.

Information concerning the efficiency of processes in preventing exposures (e.g. drip irrigation, withholding periods and other health protection measures) combined with data on the occurrence of pathogens and chemicals in wastewaters allow for the definition of operating conditions that would reasonably be expected to achieve the health-based targets (see chapter 4). Information on process efficiency and pathogen occurrence should take account of steady-state performance and performance during maintenance and periods of unusual load. While the indicator systems required to verify adequate performance may require the use of laboratory-based analytical measures (e.g. for *E. coli* or helminth egg analysis), relatively greater emphasis should be given to periodic inspection and simple analytical tests providing rapid results to inform system operation. External supervision of the system is an important feature to ensure that the system is working as described and that regulations are complied with (see chapter 6) (Bartram, Fewtrell & Stenström, 2001).

2.7 Public health status

Section 2.2 identifies different hazards associated with wastewater use in agriculture. The hazards most likely to cause disease are the excreta-related pathogens (including the intestinal helminths and schistosomes), skin irritants and vector-borne pathogens. Risks from most chemicals are thought to be low and would be difficult to associate with exposure through wastewater use in agriculture because of the long exposure times required to cause illnesses in most cases. Table 2.4 illustrates examples of mortality and morbidity estimates for some diseases of possible relevance to wastewater use in agriculture.

Table 2.4 Global mortality and DALYs due to some diseases of relevance to wastewater use in agriculture

Disease	Mortality (deaths/year)	Burden of disease (DALYs/year)	Comments
Diarrhoea	1 798 000	61 966 000	99.8% of deaths occur in developing countries; 90% of deaths occur in children
Typhoid	600 000	N/A	Estimated 16 million cases per year
Schistosomiasis	15 000	1 702 000	Found in 74 countries; 200 million people worldwide are estimated to be infected, 20 million with severe consequences
Ascariasis	3 000	1 817 000	Estimated 1.45 billion infections, of which 350 million suffer adverse health effects
Hookworm disease	3 000	59 000	Estimated 1.3 billion infections, of which 150 million suffer adverse health effects
Lymphatic filariasis	0	5 777 000	Mosquito vectors of filariasis breed in organically polluted water; does not cause death but leads to severe disability
Hepatitis A	N/A	N/A	Estimated 1.4 million cases per year worldwide; serological evidence of prior infection ranges from 15% to nearly 100%

N/A, not available
Sources: WHO (2000c, 2002, 2003b, 2003c, 2004b).

2.7.1 Excreta-related diseases

Excreta-related infections (see Table 2.5) are communicable diseases whose causative agents (pathogenic viruses, bacteria, protozoa and helminths) are released from the bodies of infected persons (or animals in some cases) in their excreta (faeces, urine). The causative agents eventually reach other people and enter either via the mouth (e.g. when contaminated crops are eaten) or via the skin (e.g. hookworm infection and schistosomiasis). The diseases of most relevance differ from area to area, depending on the general status of sanitation and hygiene in an area and the level to which wastewater is treated prior to use in agriculture. In places where hygiene and sanitary standards are poor, intestinal helminths frequently pose the greatest health risks.

Table 2.5 Excreta-related diseases

Agent	Disease
Bacteria	
Campylobacter jejuni	Gastroenteritis, long-term sequelae (e.g. arthritis)
Escherichia coli	Gastroenteritis
E. coli O157:H7	Bloody diarrhoea, haemolytic uraemic syndrome
Leptospira spp.	Leptospirosis
Salmonella (many serotypes)	Salmonellosis, gastroenteritis, diarrhoea, long-term sequelae (e.g. arthritis)
Salmonella typhi	Typhoid fever
Shigella (several serotypes)	Shigellosis (dysentery), long-term sequelae (e.g. arthritis)
Vibrio cholerae	Cholera
Yersinia enterocolitica	Yersiniosis, gastroenteritis, diarrhoea, long-term sequelae (e.g. arthritis)
Helminths	
Ancylostoma duodenale and *Necator americanus* (hookworm)	Hookworm infection
Ascaris lumbricoides (roundworm)	Ascariasis
Clonorchis sinensis (liver fluke)	Clonorchiasis
Diphyllobothrium latum (fish tapeworm)	Diphyllobothriasis
Fasciola hepatica and *F. gigantica* (liver fluke)	Fascioliasis
Fasciolopsis buski (intestinal fluke)	Fasciolopsiasis
Opisthorchis viverrini (liver fluke)	Opisthorchiasis
Paragonimus westermani (lung fluke)	Paragonimiasis
Schistosoma spp. (blood fluke)	Schistosomiasis, bilharzia[a]
Taenia saginata and *T. solium* (tapeworm)	Taeniasis
Trichuris trichuria (whipworm)	Trichuriasis
Protozoa	
Balantidium coli	Balantidiasis (dysentery)
Cryptosporidium parvum	Cryptosporidiosis, diarrhoea, fever
Cyclospora cayetanensis	Persistent diarrhoea
Entamoeba histolytica	Amoebiasis (amoebic dysentery)
Giardia intestinalis	Giardiasis

Table 2.5 (continued)

Agent	Disease
Viruses	
Adenovirus (many types)	Respiratory disease, eye infections
Astrovirus (many types)	Gastroenteritis
Calicivirus (several types)	Gastroenteritis
Coronavirus	Gastroenteritis
Coxsackievirus A	Herpangina, aseptic meningitis, respiratory illness
Coxsackievirus B	Fever, paralysis, respiratory, heart and kidney disease
Echovirus	Fever, rash, respiratory and heart disease, aseptic meningitis
Enteroviruses (many types)	Gastroenteritis, various
Hepatitis A virus	Infectious hepatitis
Hepatitis E virus	Infectious hepatitis
Norovirus	Gastroenteritis
Parvovirus (several types)	Gastroenteritis
Poliovirus	Paralysis, aseptic meningitis
Reovirus (several types)	Not clearly established
Rotavirus (several types)	Gastroenteritis

Sources: Sagik, Moor & Sorber (1978); Hurst, Benton & Stetler (1989); Edwards (1992); National Research Council (1998).

[a] See also section 2.7.2.

In many countries, excreta-related infections are common, and excreta and wastewater contain correspondingly high concentrations of pathogens. The failure to properly treat and manage wastewater and excreta worldwide is directly responsible for adverse health and environmental effects. Human excreta have been implicated in the transmission of many infectious diseases, including cholera, typhoid, hepatitis, polio, schistosomiasis and infections by helminths (e.g. *Ascaris*, hookworms, tapeworms). Most of these excreta-related illnesses occur in children living in poor countries. Overall, WHO estimates that diarrhoea alone is responsible for 3.2% of all deaths and 4.2% of overall disease burden expressed in DALYs worldwide (WHO, 2004b). In addition to diarrhoea, WHO estimates that each year, 16 million people contract typhoid and over 1 billion people suffer from intestinal helminth infections (see Table 2.4).

Diarrhoea or gastrointestinal disease is often used as a proxy for waterborne infectious diseases. Mead et al. (1999) estimated that the average person (including all age groups) in the United States of America suffers from 0.79 episode of acute gastroenteritis (characterized by diarrhoea, vomiting or both) per year. The rates of acute gastroenteritis among adults worldwide are generally within the same order of magnitude (Table 2.6). However, children — especially those living in high-risk situations, where poor hygiene, sanitation and water quality prevail — generally have a higher rate of gastrointestinal illness. Kosek, Bern & Guerrant (2003) found that children under the age of five in developing countries experienced a median of 3.2 episodes of diarrhoea per year.

Table 2.6 Diarrhoeal disease incidence per person per year in 2000, by region and age

Region	Diarrhoeal disease incidence, all ages	Diarrhoeal disease incidence, 0–4 years	Diarrhoeal disease incidence, 5–80+ years
Developed regions	0.2	0.2–1.7	0.1–0.2
Developing regions	0.8–1.3	2.4–5.2	0.4–0.6
World average	0.7	3.7	0.4

Source: Adapted from Mathers et al. (2002).

2.7.2 Schistosomiasis

Schistosomiasis is an important parasitic disease in various parts of the world. It differs from other excreta-related diseases (see section 2.7.1) in that it requires certain species of aquatic or amphibian snail hosts to complete its life cycle, its distribution is limited by the presence or absence of these snails and it affects only people who are in direct contact with contaminated water or wastewater. The disease is endemic in 74 countries in the Eastern Mediterranean region and parts of Asia and the Americas, but most of the infections occur in sub-Saharan Africa. Schistosomiasis is an infection of the blood vessels draining the urinary bladder or the intestinal tract. The disease is caused by *Schistosoma haematobium, S. mansoni, S. japonicum, S. intercalatum* and *S. mekongi*. The life cycle requires replication in a snail intermediate host. Snails become infected by a larval stage of the parasite, known as a miracidium, which develops from eggs passed out in the urine or faeces of infected people. Cercariae released by the snails penetrate the skin of people in the water. Light infections may be asymptomatic, but heavier infections may lead to enlargement of the spleen or liver, blood loss and bladder cancer, depending on the parasite species.

2 7.3 Vector-borne diseases

Vector-borne diseases such as malaria and lymphatic filariasis are not specifically associated with the use of wastewater, but they should be considered among possible health risks in endemic areas. As part of the planning of water resource development and management projects (including wastewater irrigation projects), a health impact assessment should be conducted (see Annex 3) (WHO, 2000b). As Table 2.7 indicates, activities related to some wastewater irrigation activities could increase the population of disease vectors. However, only certain mosquitoes, especially the vectors of filariasis (e.g. *Culex quinquefasciatus*), can breed in organically polluted water. There have been reports from Pakistan about malaria vector breeding at the cleaner end of a chain of wastewater stabilization ponds. A variety of measures to reduce the breeding of vectors in wastewater use programmes are described in chapter 5.

2.7.4 Measuring public health status

The impacts of risk management actions can be measured only if the baseline health status of the affected population is known or can be approximated. Similarly, tolerable risk and health-based targets can be set only with some knowledge of:

- the incidence and prevalence of disease in the community;
- the types of diseases that may result from the use of wastewater;
- the vulnerability of different subsections of the population (e.g. people with reduced immune function or those susceptible to specific hazards).

Table 2.7 Vector-borne diseases of possible relevance to wastewater use in agriculture

Disease	Vector	Relative risk of wastewater use in agriculture	Comments
Dengue	*Aedes aegypti*	Low	Vectors breed in standing water (e.g. tires, cans, bottles, etc.). Present in South-east Asia but not China.
Filariasis	*Culex quinquefasciatus*	Medium	Vectors breed in organically polluted water. Endemic in many countries where wastewater use in agriculture is practised.
Japanese encephalitis	*Culex* spp.	Medium	Vectors breed in flooded rice fields. Endemic in many countries where wastewater use in agriculture is practised.
Malaria	*Anopheles* spp.	Low	Vectors breed in uncontaminated water; 90% of malaria cases occur in Africa. *Anopheles* breeding has been reported from serial waste stabilization ponds.

Sources: WHO (1988); TDR (2004).

It is important to understand the role that wastewater plays in the transmission of water-related disease in a community. For example, studies in Mexico indicated that a very high percentage of the Ascaris infections and diarrhoea in certain exposed communities was due to the use of wastewater in agriculture. Reducing the exposures to the pathogens in the wastewater by improving wastewater treatment had a significant impact on the improvement of public health (Cifuentes, 1998; Cifuentes et al., 2000a). If only a small proportion of water-associated ill health in a specific community can be attributed to the use of wastewater in agriculture, however (e.g. if the main route of transmission is through drinking-water), then it is not cost-effective to invest limited resources in measures intended to make that use safer. Addressing the main exposure routes first is normally more cost-effective — in this example, providing access to safe drinking-water would have a larger positive impact on public health at lower cost than building a new wastewater treatment facility.

Initial information on background levels of faecal–oral disease in the population might be based on information collected from local health-care facilities, public health surveillance, laboratory analysis, epidemiological studies or specific research conducted in a project area. Seasonal fluctuations in disease incidence should be considered — for example, rotavirus infections peak in the cold season. In evaluating the use of wastewater in a certain area, it is important to evaluate disease incidence trends. High background disease levels (e.g. intestinal worm infections) or disease outbreaks (e.g. cholera) might indicate that risk management procedures were not being implemented adequately and would need to be strengthened or reconsidered.

3

ASSESSMENT OF HEALTH RISK

Wastewater can both be a resource and present a hazard. This chapter presents the current evidence of health effects associated with the use of wastewater in agriculture from both infectious agents and chemicals. Systematic assessment of the positive health benefits of the use of wastewater in agriculture has not been conducted. The health benefits will vary in different situations. It is possible that subsistence-level farmers will benefit most from the positive health impacts in terms of food security and improved nutrition as well as be at the highest risk of negative health impacts — especially where untreated wastewater is used for irrigation.

The assessment of risk relies on two types of information: epidemiological studies and QMRA. Microbial analysis provides data for both epidemiological studies and QMRA. Each type of assessment has limitations, but, used together, they can provide complementary information (see Table 3.1). Evidence from each category is presented in this section.

Table 3.1 Data used for the assessment of health risk

Type of study	Contributions	Limitations
Microbial analysis	Determines concentrations of different excreted organisms in wastewater or on products	Expensive
	Provides data on pathogen die-off rates	Collection of samples may be time-consuming
	Information used in QMRA to assess risk	Needs trained staff and laboratory facilities
	Can help to identify sources of pathogens	Obtaining laboratory results takes time
	Used to link pathogen to infection/disease (e.g. through analysis of stool samples or detection of seropositive individuals)	Lack of standardized procedures for the detection of some pathogens or their recovery from food products
		Recovery percentages may show high variability
		Some methods do not determine viability
Epidemiological study	Measures actual disease in an exposed population	Expensive
	Can be used to test different exposure hypotheses	Bias can affect results
		Sample sizes needed to measure statistically significant health outcomes may be large
		Need to strike a balance between power of the study in relation to its sensitivity
QMRA	Can estimate very low levels of risk of infection/disease	Exposure scenarios can vary significantly and are difficult to model
	Low-cost method of predicting risk of infection/disease	Validated data inputs are not available for every exposure scenario
	Facilitates comparisons of different exposure routes	Predicts risks from exposure to one type of pathogen at a time

Epidemiological studies can determine either the excess prevalence of infection (as measured by the proportion of infected or seropositive individuals) in an exposed group compared with that in a control group or the excess prevalence or incidence of disease (occurring during a specified time period) in an exposed group compared with a control group. Epidemiological studies need to use an adequate sample size based on the:

- required level of statistical significance of the expected result;
- acceptable chance of missing a real effect;
- magnitude of the effect under investigation;
- amount of disease in the population;
- relative sizes of the groups being compared.

Generally, the larger the sample size, the more power the study has to find associations between disease and exposure factors. Sample size is determined by logistic and financial considerations, and normally a compromise has to be made between sample size and costs (Beaglehole, Bonita & Kjellström, 1993).

In the context of these Guidelines, individuals eating wastewater-irrigated salad crops, working (or playing) in wastewater-irrigated fields or living near wastewater-irrigated fields (especially where spray irrigation is used) are exposed groups, and those not meeting these criteria belong to control groups.

QMRA estimates the risk of infection in an exposed group, and this can be extended to estimate the risk of disease in that group by knowing (or making an assumption about) the likely proportion of infected individuals who develop the disease.

3.1 Microbial analysis

Microbial evidence can be used to indicate that a hazard exists in the environment. Microbial analysis is an important process for providing data for the assessment of risk. Information concerning the types and numbers of different pathogens in wastewater and on irrigated produce can be used to quantify risk. These factors will vary according to region, climate, season, etc. and thus should be measured, whenever possible, on a site-specific basis.

Untreated wastewater contains a variety of excreted organisms, including pathogens, with types and numbers that vary depending on the background levels of infection in the population. Disease outbreaks result in increased concentrations of the causative agents in the wastewater and excreta. Table 3.2 shows ranges of concentrations for different excreted organisms that may be found in wastewater. Because pathogen types and concentrations can vary over a large range, it is helpful to collect local data to evaluate risk and develop risk management strategies.

Pathogens are rarely measured directly in wastewater, because their concentrations vary and analytical procedures are often difficult or expensive to perform. Instead, indicators of faecal contamination, such as *E. coli* or thermotolerant coliforms, have been used as proxies for pathogens with similar properties that may be present in wastewater. Usually, but not always, their presence in water is proportionately related to the amount of faecal contamination present. For wastewater, indicators can show how much treatment or natural purification has taken place and thus give a rough estimate of the risk associated with its use. Standardized analytical procedures have been developed for *E. coli* and thermotolerant coliforms and are widely used.

Table 3.2 Excreted organism concentrations in wastewater

Organism	Numbers in wastewater (per litre)
Bacteria	
Thermotolerant coliforms	$10^8–10^{10}$
Campylobacter jejuni	$10–10^4$
Salmonella spp.	$1–10^5$
Shigella spp.	$10–10^4$
Vibrio cholerae	$10^2–10^5$
Helminths	
Ascaris lumbricoides	$1–10^3$
Ancylostoma duodenale / Necator americanus	$1–10^3$
Trichuris trichiura	$1–10^2$
Schistosoma mansoni	ND
Protozoa	
Cryptosporidium parvum	$1–10^4$
Entamoeba histolytica	$1–10^2$
Giardia intestinalis	$10^2–10^5$
Viruses	
Enteric viruses	$10^5–10^6$
Rotavirus	$10^2–10^5$

ND, no data

Sources: Feachem et al. (1983); Mara & Silva (1986); Oragui et al. (1987); Yates & Gerba (1998).

Unfortunately, there is no perfect indicator organism for wastewater, especially for non-faecal bacterial pathogens, helminths, viruses and protozoa, as the concentrations of faecal indicator bacteria often do not correspond to concentrations of these organisms. If the wastewater effluents have been chlorinated, this will significantly reduce the numbers of bacteria but does not reduce concentrations of viruses, protozoa or helminths to the same degree.

Table 3.3 provides some examples of indicator organisms that have been used to assess the risks associated with the use of wastewater in agriculture in different situations. However, many of these indicators have been used in research studies and are not suitable for use in routine monitoring, due to the expense incurred and the need for adequate equipment. The *E. coli*/thermotolerant coliform group of bacteria is used in most water-related guidelines, as these bacteria are the most commonly monitored of the indicators that are related to faecal contamination. For further discussion of the advantages and disadvantages of different faecal indicators, see WHO (2004a) and Jiménez (2003).

Table 3.3 Examples of indicator organisms for human pathogens in wastewaters

Human pathogen	Indicator organisms	Comment
Bacteria		
Shigella, enterotoxigenic *E. coli*, *Campylobacter*, *Vibrio cholerae* (cholera)	*E. coli*, thermotolerant coliforms, intestinal enterococci	The *E. coli* /thermotolerant coliform group of bacteria has been used for more than 100 years as a model for pathogenic bacteria. Behaviour of *E. coli* and intestinal enterococci (not total coliforms) under environmental conditions is expected to reflect enteric pathogens, but not environmental bacteria such as *Legionella or Mycobacterium.*
Viruses		
Adenovirus, rotavirus, enteroviruses, hepatitis A virus, norovirus	Bacteriophages: somatic coliphages or F-RNA coliphages	Bacteriophages are viruses that infect bacteria, are considered to be non-pathogenic to humans and can be readily cultured and enumerated in the laboratory. Generally present in faeces of warm-blooded animals, but certain strains may be specific to humans.
Protozoa		
Cryptosporidium oocysts, *Giardia* cysts	*Clostridium perfringens*	*Clostridium perfringens* is a spore-forming bacterium that is highly resistant to environmental conditions. It has been shown to be a useful model for *Cryptosporidium* oocysts and *Giardia* cysts. Aerobic (*Bacillus*) spores could also be used, but are likely to grow in treatment systems and slough off surfaces, providing misleading numbers. Because protozoa are much larger than *Clostridium* spores, they will be removed in different ways during wastewater treatment processes. Validation testing should be performed with protozoan (oo)cysts or particles that are similar in size.
Helminths		
Ascaris lumbricoides and *Trichuris trichiura* ova	*Ascaris* ova	*Ascaris* and some other helminth ova (e.g. *Trichuris, Taenia*) can be measured directly. Viability of ova can be determined.

Source: Adapted from Petterson & Ashbolt (2003).

3.1.1 Survival of pathogens in soil and on crops

Many pathogens can survive for long enough periods of time in soil or on crop surfaces to be transmitted to humans or animals. The pathogens most resistant in the environment are helminth eggs, which in some cases can survive for several years in the soil. Pathogen survival depends on a number of factors, as outlined in Table 3.4. Data on pathogen survival in soil and on different crops are presented in Table 3.5. Pathogen inactivation is much more rapid in hot, sunny weather than in cool, cloudy or rainy conditions. Low temperatures prolong pathogen survival. This is particularly relevant for post-harvest storage. If plants are harvested and then transported and stored in refrigerated conditions (e.g. 4 °C), pathogens may be able to survive long enough to infect product consumers. For example, experiments on lettuce spiked with *Cryptosporidium* oocysts showed that after three days of incubation at 20 °C, no viable oocysts could be detected, while three days at 4 °C yielded 10% viable oocysts (Warnes & Keevil, 2003). Table 3.4 also shows that pathogens die off on crops more quickly than they die off in soil. Recontamination of the crops, especially root crops and crops close to the soil, can occur — particularly after rainfall.

Table 3.4 Factors that affect pathogen survival in the environment

Factor	Comment
Humidity	Humid environments favour pathogen survival.
	Dry environments facilitate pathogen die-off.
Soil content	Clay soils and soils with high organic content favour survival of pathogens.
Temperature	Most important factor in pathogen die-off. High temperatures lead to rapid die-off, and low temperatures lead to prolonged survival. Freezing temperatures can also cause pathogen die-off.
pH	Some viruses survive longer in lower-pH soils, while alkaline soils are associated with more rapid die-off of viruses; neutral to slightly alkaline soils favour bacterial survival.
Sunlight (ultraviolet radiation)	Direct sunlight leads to rapid pathogen inactivation through desiccation and exposure to ultraviolet radiation.
Foliage/plant type	Certain plants have sticky surfaces (e.g. zucchini) or can absorb pathogens from the environment (e.g. lettuce, sprouts), leading to prolonged survival of some pathogens; root crops such as onions are more prone to contamination and facilitate pathogen survival.
Competition with native flora and fauna	Antagonistic effects from bacteria or algae may enhance die-off; bacteria may be preyed upon by protozoa.

Sources: Strauss (1985); Jimenéz (2003).

Table 3.5 Survival of various organisms in selected environmental media at 20–30 °C

Organism	Survival times (days)		
	Fresh water and sewage	Crops	Soil
Viruses			
Enteroviruses[a]	<120, usually <50	<60, usually <15	<100, usually <20
Bacteria			
Thermotolerant coliforms	<60, usually <30	<30, usually <15	<70, usually <20
Salmonella spp.	<60, usually <30	<30, usually <15	<70, usually <20
Shigella spp.	<30, usually <10	<10, usually <5	ND
V. cholerae	ND	<5, usually <2	<20, usually <10
Protozoa			
E. histolytica cysts	<30, usually <15	<10, usually <2	<20, usually <10
Cryptosporidium oocysts	<180, usually <70	<3, usually <2	<150, usually <75
Helminths			
Ascaris eggs	Years	<60, usually <30	Years
Tapeworm eggs	Many months	<60, usually <30	Many months

ND, no data

Sources: Feachem et al. (1983); Strauss (1985); Robertson, Campbell & Smith (1992); Jenkins et al. (2002); Warnes & Keevil (2003).

[a] Poliovirus, echovirus and coxsackievirus.

The greatest health risks are associated with crops that are eaten raw — for example, salad crops, especially if they are root crops (e.g. radish, onion) — or that grow close to the soil (lettuce, zucchini). Certain crops may be more susceptible to contamination than others — for example, onions (Blumenthal et al., 2003), zucchini (Armon et al., 2002) and lettuce (Solomon, Yaron & Matthews, 2002). Generally, crops that have certain surface properties (e.g. hairy, sticky, crevices, rough, etc.) protect pathogens from exposure to radiation and make them more difficult to wash off with rain or by post-harvest washing. The amount of water each crop holds is also an important factor in exposure to pathogens. For example, Shuval, Lampert & Fattal (1997) estimated that lettuce retains 10.8 ml of irrigation water, while a cucumber holds only 0.36 ml — i.e. approximately 3% of the volume of water the lettuce retains. A study by Stine et al. (2005) showed that lettuce and cantaloupe surfaces retained pathogens from irrigation water spiked with *E. coli* and a bacteriophage (PRD1), but bell peppers, which are smooth, did not.

Bacteria

A summary of the results of the selected studies on bacteria survival in crops, discussed in more detail below, is given in Table 3.6.

Table 3.6 Summary of selected microbial evidence of effect of water quality on crop contamination with bacteria

Treatment type and effluent quality; thermotolerant coliforms/100 ml	Summary of evidence	Reference
Trickling filter; 10^6	The lettuces irrigated in uncovered plots had high levels of bacterial contamination, unless a period of cessation of irrigation occurred before harvest (e.g. 7–12 days).	Vas da Costa Vargas, Bastos & Mara (1996)
Waste stabilization pond; 10^3–10^4	The quality of irrigated radishes and lettuces was 10^3 and 10^4 *E. coli* per 100 g (worst case) in dry weather; contamination increased after rainfall, and *Salmonella* bacteria were isolated.	Bastos & Mara (1995)
(i) Wastewater storage reservoir; 10^7; (ii) wastewater storage reservoir; 10^2	Improving the water quality to 200 thermotolerant coliforms/100 ml improved the quality of vegetables from 10^5 to <10^3 thermotolerant coliforms/100 ml.	Armon et al. (1994)
(i) Raw wastewater; 10^7; (ii) waste stabilization pond; 10^5; (iii) river water; 10^2	The percentage of crops with detectable salmonella decreased as water quality increased; leafy salad crops growing near the soil were the most contaminated; cessation of irrigation 8 days before harvest improved crop quality.	Castro de Esparza & Vargas (1990, cited in Peasy et al., 2000)

Studies in Portugal (Vaz da Costa Vargas, Bastos & Mara, 1996) showed that when a poor-quality wastewater (trickling filter effluent with 10^6 thermotolerant coliforms per 100 ml) was used to spray-irrigate lettuces, initial concentrations of indicator bacteria exceeded 10^5 thermotolerant coliforms per 100 g fresh weight. Once irrigation ceased, no *Salmonella* could be detected after five days, and after 7–12 days, thermotolerant coliform levels were similar to or just above the level seen in lettuces irrigated with fresh water. The crop quality was better than that of lettuces irrigated with surface waters on sale in the local markets (10^6 thermotolerant coliforms per 100 g), presumably because of recontamination in the market through the use of contaminated freshening water.

Studies of drip and furrow irrigation of lettuces and radishes (Bastos & Mara, 1995) with waste stabilization pond effluent (1700–5000 thermotolerant coliforms per 100 ml) indicated that crop quality was better under dry weather conditions: 10^3 and 10^4 *E. coli* per 100 g for radishes and lettuces and no *Salmonella* was present. The crop quality was better than that of locally sold lettuces (10^6 *E. coli* per 100 g). However, when rainfall occurred, *E. coli* numbers increased, and *Salmonella* bacteria were isolated from lettuce surfaces

Studies in Israel (Armon et al., 1994) showed that, when vegetables and salad crops were irrigated with poor-quality effluent from wastewater storage reservoirs (up to 10^7 thermotolerant coliforms per 100 ml), high levels of faecal indicator bacteria were detected on crop surfaces (up to 10^5 thermotolerant coliforms per 100 ml). However, when vegetables were irrigated with better-quality effluent (0–200 thermotolerant coliforms per 100 ml) from a different storage reservoir, thermotolerant coliform levels on crops were generally $<10^3$ per 100 g and often lower. In Peru, Castro de Esparza & Vargas (1990, cited in Peasy et al., 2000) found that the percentage of crops with detectable *Salmonella* decreased as water quality improved, from 10^7 thermotolerant coliforms in raw wastewater (10^3 *Salmonella* per 100 ml) to 10^5 thermotolerant coliforms ($<10^2$ *Salmonella*) in treated effluent from a wastewater stabilization pond. No *Salmonella* was detected on crops irrigated with river water (200 thermotolerant coliforms and no *Salmonella* detected). The most contaminated crop was lettuce, followed by parsley, spinach and carrots. Allowing eight days between the last irrigation and harvest ensured a 25% increase in crop samples having <10 *E. coli* and no detectable *Salmonella* per gram.

Overall, these studies indicate that (i) irrigating salad crops with wastewater containing $>10^5$ thermotolerant coliforms per 100 ml in uncovered plots results in high levels of bacterial contamination of crops, unless a period of cessation of irrigation occurs before harvest; (ii) improving the quality to 10^2–10^3 thermotolerant coliforms per 100 ml results in crops with low levels of contamination ($<10^3$ thermotolerant coliforms per 100 ml); and (iii) crop recontamination occurs frequently in markets.

Helminths

A summary of the data presented in this section is given in Table 3.7.

Table 3.7 Summary of selected microbial evidence of effect of water quality on crop contamination with helminths

Treatment type and effluent quality; number of nematode eggs per litre	Summary of evidence	Reference
(i) Raw wastewater; >100	Lettuce contamination levels at harvest were:	Ayres et al. (1992a)
(ii) Waste stabilization pond; >10	(i) up to 60 eggs/plant	
(iii) Waste stabilization pond; <0.5	(ii) 0.6 egg/plant	
(iv) Waste stabilization pond; 0	(iii) 0 eggs/plant	
	(iv) 0 eggs/plant	
(i) Waste stabilization pond; 50	Lettuce contamination levels at harvest were:	Stott et al. (1994)
(ii) Waste stabilization pond; 10	(i) up to 2.2 eggs/plant	
(iii) Waste stabilization pond; ≤1	(ii) maximum 1.5 eggs/plant	
	(iii) 0.3 egg/plant	

Studies in Brazil (Ayres et al., 1992a) indicated that when lettuce was spray-irrigated with effluent from waste stabilization ponds, the levels of crop contamination decreased with increased pond retention time, from the anaerobic pond through to the maturation pond. Levels of nematode contamination of lettuce were 0.6 egg per plant at harvest from the anaerobic pond (>10 eggs per litre), and no nematode eggs were detected on lettuces irrigated with effluent from the facultative pond (<0.5 egg per litre) or the maturation pond (0 eggs per litre, i.e. eggs were not detectable), despite growing in heavily contaminated soil containing >1200 *Ascaris* eggs per 100 g. Irrigation with fresh water successfully removed small levels of contamination on crops, whereas rainfall events significantly reduced levels of contamination on crops.

Studies carried out in greenhouses in the United Kingdom (Stott et al., 1994) with seeded effluent (*Ascaridia galli*) indicated that irrigation with wastewater containing 10 eggs per litre resulted in low levels of nematode contamination on lettuce (maximum of 1.5 eggs per plant), and improving wastewater quality further to ≤1 egg per litre resulted in very slight contamination of some plants (0.3 egg per plant). However, no transmission of *A. galli* infection was found from wastewater-irrigated crops using animal studies, although the infective dose was very low at <5 embryonated eggs.

The collective outcome of these microbial analyses shows that irrigation with wastewater at a quality of ≤1 egg per litre results in no detectable contamination of lettuce at harvest or at most only a very slight contamination on some plants (6%) with eggs that were either degenerate or not infective. However, a few nematode eggs on harvested plants were viable but not yet embryonated, indicating that crops with a long shelf life could represent a potential risk to consumers if the eggs had sufficient time to become infective.

Protozoa

In general, limited evidence concerning crop contamination with protozoa resulting from wastewater irrigation is available. Armon et al. (2002) found that zucchini spray-irrigated with poor-quality wastewater (>100 oocysts per litre) accumulated higher levels of *Cryptosporidium* oocysts (80–10 000 oocysts per 0.5 kg) on the surface than other types of crops. Zucchini have hairy, sticky surfaces and grow close to the ground and therefore may concentrate certain types of pathogens on the surface.

In Peru, *Entamoeba coli* was the most common protozoan and was identified on 38% of crops irrigated with wastewater and other contaminated surface water sources (Castro de Esparza & Vargas, 1990, cited in Peasey et al., 2000). *Cryptosporidium* and *Cyclospora* oocysts have been identified on produce sold in markets in Peru (Ortega et al., 1997) and Costa Rica (Calvo et al., 2004). In these cases, no water quality data were available, and contamination was more likely to have been caused by the use of sewage-contaminated surface water for irrigation rather than the direct use of wastewater for irrigation. The presence of *Cyclospora cayetanensis* in wastewater from the area where crops were produced in Peru has been confirmed by Sturbaum et al. (1998).

Viruses

A number of studies concerning viral die-off on crops have been conducted. In general, survival of viruses is influenced by the same parameters as described in Table 3.4. Petterson et al. (2001a) modelled the inactivation of enteric viruses on lettuce and carrots using data collected on crops grown under greenhouse conditions

Table 3.8 Viral inactivation on different crops

Crops	T[99] (days)	Data source	References
Artichoke, broccoli, celery and lettuce	1.45	Seeded poliovirus inactivation over four days in an environmental chamber	Engineering Science (1987); Asano et al. (1992)
Celery (environmental chamber)	1.82[a]	Poliovirus seeded onto plants and time for 99% removal were recorded in both an environmental chamber and under field conditions	Sheikh, Cooper & Israel (1999)
Iceberg lettuce (environmental chamber)	3.3[a]		
Romaine lettuce (field conditions)	1.25[a]		
Butter lettuce (field conditions)	1.7[a]		
Winter triumph lettuce	0.4 (fast phase) 2 (slow phase) subpopulation size 0.12%[b]	Plants spray-irrigated at maturity with wastewater seeded with *B. fragilis* bacteriophage B40-8; experiment undertaken in uncontrolled greenhouse conditions	Petterson et al. (2001b)
Carrot	1.25 (fast phase) 20 (slow phase) subpopulation size 2%[b]	Plants grown in pots and irrigated at maturity with wastewater seeded with *B. fragilis* bacteriophage B40-8; experiment undertaken in uncontrolled greenhouse conditions	Petterson et al. (2001b)

T[99], time required for a 99% (2-log) reduction
[a] Estimated value of inactivation coefficient assuming log-linear relationship ($C_t = C_0 e^{-ht}$) and time for 2 log virus removal. Added here for the purpose of comparison; not included in cited paper.
[b] The data showed evidence of biphasic decay (Petterson et al., 2001b).

and irrigated with wastewater seeded with a model virus *Bacteroides fragilis* B40-8. The results showed evidence for biphasic inactivation and notably the presence of a persistent subpopulation of viruses. Ward & Irving (1987) observed survival times of 1–13 days when the irrigation water contained between 5.1×10^2 and 2.6×10^5 type 1 poliovirus VU per litre.

Most of the studies conducted with viruses have been based on wastewater or water seeded with viruses. However, Hernandez et al. (1997) found hepatitis A viruses and rotaviruses in market lettuce irrigated with contaminated water in Costa Rica.

Table 3.8 illustrates some experimentally determined viral inactivation rates on different types of vegetables (Petterson & Ashbolt, 2003).

3.2 Epidemiological evidence

Shuval et al. (1986) conducted a review of the available epidemiological evidence from studies of wastewater use in agriculture. The evidence at that time suggested that the use of untreated wastewater in agriculture presented a high risk of transmission of intestinal nematodes and bacterial infections, especially to produce consumers and farm workers; there was limited evidence that the health of people living near wastewater-irrigated fields was affected. There was less evidence for the transmission of viruses and no evidence for the transmission of parasitic protozoa to farm workers,

Table 3.9 Summary of health risks associated with the use of wastewater for irrigation

Group exposed	Health risks		
	Helminth infections	Bacterial/virus infections	Protozoal infections
Consumers	Significant risk of helminth infection for both adults and children with untreated wastewater	Cholera, typhoid and shigellosis outbreaks reported from use of untreated wastewater; seropositive responses for *Helicobacter pylori* (untreated); increase in non-specific diarrhoea when water quality exceeds 10^4 thermotolerant coliforms/100 ml	Evidence of parasitic protozoa found on wastewater-irrigated vegetable surfaces, but no direct evidence of disease transmission
Farm workers and their families	Significant risk of helminth infection for both adults and children in contact with untreated wastewater; increased risk of hookworm infection for workers who do not wear shoes; risk for helminth infection remains, especially for children, even when wastewater is treated to <1 helminth egg per litre; adults are not at increased risk at this helminth concentration	Increased risk of diarrhoeal disease in young children with wastewater contact if water quality exceeds 10^4 thermotolerant coliforms/100 ml; elevated risk of *Salmonella* infection in children exposed to untreated wastewater; elevated seroresponse to norovirus in adults exposed to partially treated wastewater	Risk of *Giardia intestinalis* infection reported to be insignificant for contact with both untreated and treated wastewater; however, another study in Pakistan has estimated a threefold increase in risk of *Giardia* infection for farmers using raw wastewater compared with irrigation with fresh water; increased risk of amoebiasis observed with contact with untreated wastewater
Nearby communities	Transmission of helminth infections not studied for sprinkler irrigation, but same as above for flood or furrow irrigation with heavy contact	Sprinkler irrigation with poor water quality (10^6–10^8 total coliforms/100 ml) and high aerosol exposure associated with increased rates of infection; use of partially treated water (10^4–10^5 thermotolerant coliforms/100 ml or less) in sprinkler irrigation is not associated with increased viral infection rates	No data on transmission of protozoan infections during sprinkler irrigation with wastewater

Sources: Shuval, Yekutiel & Fattal (1984); Fattal et al. (1986); Shuval et al. (1989); Blumenthal et al. (2000a); Armon et al. (2002); Blumenthal & Peasey (2002); J.H.J. Ensink, W. van der Hoek & F.P. Amerasinghe (unpublished data, 2005).

consumers or nearby communities. The evidence also indicated that irrigation with treated wastewater did not lead to excess intestinal nematode infections among fieldworkers or consumers. The information from this review informed the development of the second edition of the WHO Guidelines (WHO, 1989).

Blumenthal & Peasey (2002) completed a critical review of all the epidemiological evidence of the health effects of wastewater and excreta use in agriculture for WHO. A summary of the main epidemiological evidence is presented in the following section, which has been abstracted from Blumenthal & Peasey (2002), and further summarized in Table 3.9 (summarized in Carr, Blumenthal & Mara, 2004). For studies where prevalence data were reported, a crude relative risk and 95% confidence interval were calculated where there was no calculation of a measure of association between exposure and infection. In the summary tables (see Tables 3.10–3.13 below), significance levels were reported using *P*-values at three levels ($P < 0.05$ denoted by *, $P < 0.01$ denoted by **, $P < 0.001$ denoted by ***). In the original study, studies were then evaluated according to their epidemiological quality, where analytical studies were better than descriptive studies, prospective studies better than retrospective studies and cohort studies better than cross-sectional studies. Most credence was given to a subset of analytical epidemiological studies that included the following features: well defined exposure and disease, risk estimates calculated after allowance for confounding factors, statistical testing of associations between exposure and disease and evidence of causality (where available). These studies are given more prominence in the text, and the overall results reported for each section give more credence to the results from these analytical studies.

3.2.1 Risks to consumers of crops eaten uncooked

Table 3.10 (pages 36-37) summarizes the studies that were reviewed on risks of helminth, bacterial and viral infections to consumers of crops eaten uncooked. The results of comparison of exposed and non-exposed groups are given as relative risks or odds ratios in the table (ratio of exposed to non-exposed) and reported as attributable risks in the text (difference between exposed and non-exposed).

Helminth infections

Descriptive studies (Khalil, 1931; Baumhogger, 1949; Krey, 1949; Shuval, Yekutiel & Fattal, 1984) of the association between consumption of uncooked vegetables irrigated with untreated wastewater and *Ascaris* infection produced estimates of relative risks between 7.0 and 35.0 (Table 3.10); the proportion of *Ascaris* infection in the study populations that was attributed to consumption of uncooked vegetables irrigated with wastewater (the attributable risk) varied between 34% and 60%. An analytical cross-sectional study (Cifuentes, 1998) provided an estimate of relative risk of 1.4, but it is not clear how much this is a measure of the risk of the use of untreated or treated wastewater, as stratum-specific estimates were not reported.

A prospective cohort study (Peasey, 2000), however, produced adjusted odds ratios (OR) of 3.9 (men) and 2.4 (children) for consumption of vegetables irrigated with wastewater by farming families, when allowance was made for potential confounding factors for *Ascaris* such as age, gender, socioeconomic status and direct wastewater contact. The attributable risk from consumption was 25% for children and 14% for adult men. The proportion of infection in the whole study population that was attributable to exposure and could be eliminated if the exposure were removed (the preventable fraction) was 53% and 35% for children and adult men, respectively.

There is some evidence in adult men that consumption of vegetables irrigated with untreated wastewater (>100 eggs per litre) had a greater effect than irrigation with treated wastewater (<1 egg per litre) (OR = 2.7, $P = 0.074$ and OR = 0.6, $P = 0.68$, respectively), but this did not reach statistical significance. In children, irrigation of vegetables with untreated wastewater was associated with an increased risk of infection (OR = 4.2, $P < 0.001$), and use of treated wastewater (<1 nematode egg per litre) was also associated with an increased risk of infection (OR = 3.7, $P = 0.056$). A descriptive (ecological) study (Baumhogger, 1949; Krey, 1949) provides suggestive evidence that treatment using sedimentation and biological oxidation reduces the risks of *Ascaris* among consumers of uncooked vegetables to below the levels seen where no wastewater irrigation takes place.

Bacterial and viral infections

There are several studies of the risk of specific bacterial or viral infections associated with consumption of vegetable crops irrigated with untreated wastewater. A study in Santiago, Chile (Hopkins et al., 1993) showed that the consumption of raw vegetables coming from an area where untreated wastewater is used for irrigation was related to an increase in seroprevalence to *Helicobacter pylori* (relative risk 3.3, $P < 0.001$), when allowance was made for confounding factors.

Analytical cross-sectional studies of symptomatic diarrhoeal disease in Mexico (Blumenthal et al., 2003) indicated that there was a twofold or greater risk of diarrhoeal disease associated with medium or high frequencies of consumption of uncooked onions irrigated with wastewater that had been stored in a single reservoir (water quality 10^4 thermotolerant coliforms per 100 ml). For adults, the attributable risk was 4.3% (weekly prevalence), which is equivalent to an annual rate of 0.66 per person (allowing for an eight-month dry season). A prospective cohort study in the same area showed that there was a twofold increase in seroresponse to norovirus (Mexico strain) associated with the consumption of green tomatoes irrigated with the same water when allowance was made for confounding factors, but no increased risk of seroresponse to enterotoxigenic *E. coli* infection associated with vegetable consumption. In this study, over 50% of the diarrhoeal disease in the study population who ate onions (which was over half the study group) was attributable to consumption of onions, such that over 25% of all diarrhoea in adults and young children in the study population in the dry season was attributable to wastewater irrigation of vegetables.

Evidence from disease outbreaks

Study of disease outbreaks provides further information on risks to consumers from irrigating vegetables with wastewater. From disease outbreaks in Chile and Israel, there is evidence of the transmission of cholera (Shuval, Yekutiel & Fattal, 1984; Fattal, Yekutiel & Shuval, 1986), typhoid (Shuval, 1993) and shigellosis (Porter et al., 1984) when vegetables are irrigated with untreated wastewater.

Summary

There is evidence to suggest that the use of untreated wastewater to irrigate vegetables can lead to increased helminth infection (mainly *Ascaris lumbricoides* infection), bacterial and viral infections (typhoid, cholera, *Helicobacter pylori*, norovirus) and symptomatic diarrhoeal disease in consumers. The studies of *Ascaris* infection among consumers indicate that treatment is needed to reduce the risk of *Ascaris* infection to consumers of crops irrigated with untreated wastewater. It is not possible to determine the extent of treatment that is needed from the available data, but an analytical study indicated that treatment to ≤1 nematode egg per litre may not be sufficient in certain circumstances, especially where children are exposed. When wastewater is partially treated, there is evidence that the risk of enteric infections (bacterial and viral origin) is still significant when consumers eat some types of uncooked vegetables (mainly root crops) irrigated by water with 10^4 thermotolerant coliforms per 100 ml.

3.2.2 Risks to agricultural workers and their families

Table 3.11 summarizes the studies that were reviewed on risks of transmission of intestinal parasitic infections to agricultural workers, their families and nearby populations. Table 3.12 summarizes the studies that were reviewed on the prevalence of reported enteric disease in agricultural workers, their families and nearby populations. Table 3.13 summarizes the serological studies that were reviewed on risks of transmission of enteric viruses and bacteria to agricultural workers and nearby populations.

Research conducted in Phnom Penh, Cambodia, indicated that there may be an association between exposure to wastewater and skin problems such as contact dermatitis (eczema) (van der Hoek et al., 2005). In a survey of households engaged in the cultivation of aquatic vegetables in a lake heavily contaminated by untreated sewage, 22% of the people living in the households reported skin problems. In a survey of similar households living around a lake with no wastewater inputs, only 1% of the people reported skin problems. Skin problems were most likely to be reported on the hands (56%), feet (36%) and legs (34%). The cause of the skin problems was not determined but was likely due to a mixture of agents (i.e. both chemical and biological) in the wastewater.

Intestinal parasitic infections

There is evidence to suggest that direct contact with untreated wastewater can lead to increased helminth infection (mainly *Ascaris* and hookworm infection) and that this effect is more pronounced in children than in adult farm workers. When flood or furrow irrigation with wastewater is used, the effect of direct contact with untreated wastewater on *Ascaris* infection varies according to area and the initial prevalence, from attributable risks of between 9% and 30% in children (Bouhoum & Schwartzbrod, 1998; Habbari et al., 2000; Peasey, 2000; Blumenthal et al., 2001) and between 7% and 33% in adults (Krishnamoorthi, Abdulappa & Anwikar, 1973; Cifuentes, 1998; Peasey, 2000; Blumenthal et al., 2001). For hookworm infection, the effect of exposure to untreated wastewater among farm workers varies from attributable risks of between 37% (Krishnamoorthi, Abdulappa & Anwikar, 1973) and 14% (Ensink et al., 2005) in adults.

There is some evidence from analytical studies that *Ascaris* infection can be reduced when wastewater is partially treated before use, but the effect depends on the extent of treatment. In studies in Mexico, where wastewater retention was ensured in a single reservoir for a minimum of one month during the year preceding the study (achieving 2 log nematode egg removal, to <1 nematode egg per litre), there was no increased risk of *Ascaris* infection in adults associated with exposure to wastewater irrigation (Peasey, 2000); in children, however, there was still a significant increased attributable risk of 14% (Peasey, 2000; Blumenthal et al., 2001). However, retention in two reservoirs in series for a period of one or two months in each reservoir (achieving a 2–3 log nematode egg removal) resulted in no detected excess risk of *Ascaris* in children (Cifuentes, 1998).

There are very few data on the effect of contact with wastewater in agriculture on protozoan infections. Studies in India (Sehgal & Mahajan, 1991) and Mexico (Cifuentes et al., 2000b) have produced similar results; that is, there is no significant risk of *Giardia intestinalis* infection related to contact with untreated or treated wastewater for irrigation. However, a study in Pakistan estimated a threefold increase in risk of *Giardia* infection when farmers using raw wastewater were compared with farmers using regular (non-wastewater) irrigation water (J.H.J. Ensink, W. van der Hoek & F.P. Amerasinghe, unpublished data, 2005). The attributable risk was 28%.

Table 3.10 Studies of risks to consumers: Prevalence of infection and relative risks or odds ratios in populations consuming or not consuming uncooked vegetables irrigated with wastewater

Health outcome and outcome measure	Wastewater quality	Age group (years)	Prevalence of outcome measure (%)	Relative risk or odds ratio (95% CI)	Study group and comparison	Reference
Ascariasis (prevalence)	Untreated	Adults	70 vs 10	7.0[b]	Prison population eating vegetables irrigated with wastewater vs village population not using wastewater or nightsoil in agriculture	Khalil (1931)[a]
Ascariasis (prevalence — routine data)	Untreated	All ages	50 vs 6	8.3[b]	City where untreated wastewater used to irrigate vegetables vs average of five cities with no wastewater irrigation	Baumhogger (1949); Krey (1949)[a]
Ascariasis (prevalence — routine data)	Untreated	All ages	(i) 35 vs 1 (ii) 13 vs 1	(i) 35.0 (32.56–37.62)[b] (ii) 13.0[b]	General population eating wastewater-irrigated vegetables vs general population not consuming wastewater-irrigated vegetables (i) 1935–1947 vs 1948–1966 (ii) 1968–1970 vs 1975–1982	Shuval, Yekutiel & Fattal (1984)
Ascariasis (prevalence)	Untreated and treated (storage reservoirs)	5+	4.9 vs 2.9	1.43 (1.07–1.92)**	Consumption of local vegetables (wastewater-irrigated fields) vs vegetables grown outside village	Cifuentes (1998)
Ascariasis (prevalence)	(i) Untreated and treated (ii) Untreated (iii) Treated <1 nematode egg per litre	<15	(i) 41.1 vs 16.4 (ii) 46.5 vs 17.3 (iii) 36.5 vs 13.3	(i) 2.41 (1.07–5.44)* (ii) 4.15 (1.89–9.41)c*** (iii) 3.74 (0.80–17.38)	Consumption of uncooked vegetables from local (wastewater-irrigated) field or garden vs no consumption	Peasey (2000)
		>15 male	(i) 22.4 vs 8.8 (ii) 22.4 vs 9.5 (iii) 8.0 vs 12.5	(i) 3.93 (1.01–15.24) (ii) 2.74 (0.84–8.81) (iii) 0.61 (0.06–5.81)		
Ascariasis (prevalence)	Treated (sedimentation and biological oxidation)	All ages	2.2 vs 6.1	0.36[b]	City where treated wastewater used to irrigate vegetables vs average of five cities with no wastewater irrigation	Baumhogger (1949); Krey (1949)[a]

Table 3.10 (continued)

Health outcome and outcome measure	Wastewater quality	Age group (years)	Prevalence of outcome measure (%)	Relative risk or odds ratio (95% CI)	Study group and comparison	Reference
Helicobacter pylori infection (seroprevalence)	Untreated	<35	38 vs 9	3.25 (1.94–5.71)***	Consumption of uncooked vs cooked vegetables	Hopkins et al. (1993)
Diarrhoeal disease (self-reported two-weekly prevalence)	Untreated and treated	5+	19.0 vs 10.0	2.00 (1.37–2.93)***	Family grows salad crops (wastewater irrigated) vs family does not grow salad crops	Cifuentes (1998)
Diarrhoeal disease (self-reported weekly prevalence)	Treated (storage reservoirs); 10^4 faecal coliforms/100 ml	1–4	<1/week, 2.6 1/week, 9.5 >1/week, 5.8	1.00 3.80 (1.24–11.68) 2.19 (0.54–8.89) $P = 0.05$	Medium and high frequencies of consumption of uncooked onions vs low frequency	Blumenthal et al. (2003)
		15+	<1/month, 2.4 1–3/month, 8.7 1/week, 6.0 >1/week, 5.5	1.00 3.99 (1.62–9.82) 2.58 (1.05–6.39) 2.24 (0.88–5.71) $P < 0.01$		
Norovirus infection (Mexico strain) (seroresponse)	Treated (storage reservoirs); 10^4 faecal coliforms/100 ml	5–14	0/2 weeks, 13.6 1/2 weeks, 20.6 2–14/2 weeks, 29.6	1.00 1.44 (0.76–2.75) 2.52 (1.03–6.13)	Different frequencies of consumption of uncooked green tomatoes	Blumenthal et al. (2003)

Significance levels: *, $P < 0.05$; **, $P < 0.01$; ***, $P < 0.001$

[a] Described in Shuval et al. (1986).

[b] Crude relative risk calculated from prevalence data reported.

[c] Crude odds ratios and 95% confidence intervals calculated for prevalence data reported: (i) adjusted odds ratios; (ii) and (iii) crude odds ratios.

Table 3.11 Studies of risks to workers and nearby populations: Prevalence and relative risks of parasitic infections in populations exposed or not exposed to wastewater used for irrigation

Health outcome	Wastewater quality	Age group (years)	Prevalence of infection (%)	Relative risk or odds ratio (95% CI)	Study group and comparison	Reference
(i) Ascariasis (ii) Hookworm infection	Untreated	Adults	(i) 46.8 vs 13.4 (ii) 69.7 vs 32.6	(i) 3.48 (2.69–4.51)***[b] (ii) 2.14 (1.84–2.48)***[b]	Sewage farm workers vs farm workers exposed to clean water	Krishnamoorthi, Abdulapp & Anwikar (1973)[a]
(i) Ascariasis (ii) Trichuriasis	Untreated	School children	(i) 33 vs 2 (ii) 17 vs 2	(i) 16.5[c] (ii) 8.5[c]	School children in urban area where sewage use in irrigation vs where sewage not used	Bouhoum & Schwartzbrod (1998)
Ascariasis	Untreated	7–14	35.1 vs 19.1	1.79 (1.13–2.84)*[b]	Contact with wastewater vs no contact with wastewater	Habbari et al. (2000)
(i) Parasitic infection (ii) Hookworm	Untreated, plus health protection measures	Adult	(i) 81.6 vs 26.2 (ii) 25.1 vs 7.7	(i) 3.1[c] (ii) 3.3[c]	(i) Sewage farm workers with poor personal hygiene vs good hygiene (ii) Sewage farm workers barefoot vs wearing shoes	Srivastava & Pandey (1986)
Ascariasis	(i) Untreated (ii) Treated (one storage reservoir) <1 nematode egg per litre	0–4	(i) 10.0 vs 0.6 (ii) 11.8 vs 0.6	(i) 18.01 (4.10–79.16)*** (ii) 21.22 (5.06–88.93)***	Farm workers or their children (i) in direct contact with raw wastewater vs not using wastewater for irrigation (dry season) (ii) in direct contact with wastewater stored in one reservoir vs not using wastewater for irrigation	Blumenthal et al. (2001)
		5+	(i) 7.2 vs 0.4 (ii) 4.6 vs 0.4	(i) 13.49 (6.35–28.63)*** (ii) 9.42 (4.45–19.94)***		
Ascariasis	(i) Untreated (ii) Treated (two storage reservoirs) 0 nematode eggs per litre	0–4		(i) 5.71 (2.44–13.36)*** (ii) 1.29 (0.49–3.39)	Farm workers or their children (i) in direct contact with raw wastewater vs not using wastewater for irrigation (rainy season) (ii) in direct contact with wastewater stored in two reservoirs vs not using wastewater for irrigation	Cifuentes (1998)

Table 3.11 (continued)

Health outcome	Wastewater quality	Age group (years)	Prevalence of infection (%)	Relative risk or odds ratio (95% CI)	Study group and comparison	Reference
Ascariasis *(continued)*		5+	(i) 9.1 vs 0.7 (ii) 1.5 vs 0.7	(i) 13.18 (7.51–23.12)*** (ii) 1.94 (1.01–3.71)*	Farm workers or their children	Peasey (2000)
	(i) Untreated (ii) Treated (one storage reservoir) <1 nematode egg per litre	<15	(i) 50.0 vs 30.0 (ii) 44.1 vs 30.0	(i) 1.50 (0.59–3.79) (ii) 2.61 (1.10–6.15)**	(i) in direct contact with raw wastewater vs not in direct contact with wastewater (dry season) (ii) in direct contact with wastewater stored in one reservoir vs not in direct contact with wastewater	
		>15 male	(i) 39.3 vs 9.0 (ii) 12.5 vs 9.0	(i) 5.37 (1.79–16.10)** (ii) 1.56 (0.13–18.59)	[Direct contact was through (a) play (<15 years), (b) work relating to chili production (male >15 years), (c) tending livestock in wastewater-irrigated fields (female >15 years)]	
		>15 female	(i) 37.5 vs 15.6 (ii) 3.9 vs 15.6	(i) 4.39 (1.08–17.81)* (ii) 0.70 (0.06–8.33)		
Giardiasis	(i) Untreated (ii) Treated	Not specified	(i) 12.3 vs 11.5 (ii) 15.5 vs 11.5	(i) 1.07 (0.85–1.35)[b] (ii) 1.35 (0.99–1.86)[b]	(i) General population in villages using raw wastewater for irrigation vs general population in control village not using sewage (ii) General population in villages using treated wastewater for irrigation vs general population in control village not using sewage	Sehgal & Mahajan (1991)
Giardiasis	(i) Untreated (ii) Treated (two storage reservoirs)	All ages	(i) 8.1 vs 7.8 (ii) 10.9 vs 7.8	(i) 1.01 (0.84–1.36) (ii) 1.22 (0.94–1.58)	Farm workers and their families (i) in direct contact with raw wastewater vs not using wastewater for irrigation (ii) in direct contact with wastewater stored in two reservoirs vs not using wastewater for irrigation	Cifuentes et al. (2000b)

Significance levels: *, $P < 0.05$; **, $P < 0.01$; ***, $P < 0.001$
[a] Described in Shuval et al. (1986).
[b] Relative risk and 95% confidence interval calculated from prevalence or incidence rates and population data reported.
[c] Crude relative risk calculated from prevalence or incidence data reported.

Table 3.12 Studies of risks to workers and nearby populations: Prevalence of reported enteric infections and relative risks in populations exposed or not exposed to wastewater used for irrigation

Health outcome and outcome measure	Wastewater quality	Age group (years)	Prevalence or incidence of infection (%)	Relative risk or odds ratio (95% confidence interval)	Study group and comparison	Reference
(i) Salmonellosis (ii) Shigellosis (iii) Typhoid fever (iv) Infectious hepatitis (Incidence per 100 000 population)	Treated Stabilization ponds 3–7 days retention 10^6–10^8 total coliforms/100 ml	All ages	(i) 23.4 vs 6.3 (ii) 100.2 vs 45.5 (iii) 1.16 vs 0.27 (iv) 8.8 vs 4.4	(i) 3.7 (ii) 2.2 (iii) 4.3 (iv) 2.0	Population in kibbutzim using wastewater for irrigation vs not using wastewater	Katzenelson, Buiu & Shuval (1976)
Enteric disease (Incidence per 100 person-years)	Treated Stabilization ponds 5–10 days retention 10^6–10^8 total coliforms/100 ml	(i) 0–4 (ii) 5–18 (iii) ≥19	(i) 51.8 vs 27.4 (ii) 11.2 vs 6.6 (iii) 4.7 vs 1.8	(i) 1.91 (1.30–2.80) (ii) 1.23 (0.46–3.25) (iii) 2.06 (0.69–6.16)	Comparison of enteric disease rates in kibbutzim when using wastewater for sprinkler irrigation vs when not using wastewater for irrigation, with allowance made for rate of control diseases and other factors; results from irrigation season	Fattal et al. (1986a)
Enteric disease (Incidence per 100 person-years)	Treated Stabilization ponds 5–10 days retention 10^4–10^5 total coliforms/100 ml	All ages 0–5	L 11.0 M 9.4 H 11.6 L 26.4 M 20.0 H 26.0	L 1.00[a] M 0.85 H 1.05 L 1.00 M 0.76 H 0.98	Comparison of rates in kibbutzim population with wastewater sprinkler irrigation within 300–600 m (High = H) or kibbutzim with wastewater use but no aerosols (Medium = M) vs kibbutzim with no use of wastewater (Low = L) [No excess enteric disease was seen in wastewater contact workers or their families compared with the unexposed]	Shuval et al. (1989)
Clinical illness (Incidence per worker-month)	Treated Storage lagoons (over winter)	Adults	0.54 vs 0.58	0.93[a]	Comparison of illness rates in spray irrigation workers vs road commission workers (no significant differences found with level of exposure)	Linnemann et al. (1984)

Table 3.12 (continued)

Health outcome and outcome measure	Wastewater quality	Age group (years)	Prevalence or incidence of infection (%)	Relative risk or odds ratio (95% confidence interval)	Study group and comparison	Reference
Clinical viral infections (% with infection episode in irrigation season)	Treated (summer 1982: trickling filter plant effluent 8×10^6 faecal coliforms/100 ml, 3.2 enteroviruses/100 ml; summer 1983: effluent from trickling filter plant and storage reservoirs 10^3–10^4 faecal coliforms/100 ml, 0.4 enteroviruses/100 ml)	Adults and children <13	Summer 1982 (i) 8 (ii) 8 (iii) 24 Summer 1983 (i) 0 (ii) 8 (iii) 5	$P = 0.06$ $P > 0.05$	Comparison of faecal donors with (i) low aerosol exposure (ii) medium aerosol exposure (iii) high aerosol exposure	Camann & Moore (1987)
Diarrhoeal disease (two-weekly prevalence)	(i) Untreated (ii) Treated (one storage reservoir) 10^5 faecal coliforms/100 ml	0–4	(i) 19.4 vs 13.6 (ii) 15.6 vs 13.6	(i) 1.75 (1.10–2.78)** (ii) 1.13 (0.70–1.83)	Farm workers or their children (i) in direct contact with raw wastewater vs not using wastewater for irrigation (dry season) (ii) in direct contact with wastewater stored in one reservoir vs not using wastewater for irrigation	Blumenthal et al. (2001)
		5+	(i) 7.1 vs 5.9 (ii) 8.1 vs 5.9	(i) 1.34 (1.00–1.78)* (ii) 1.50 (1.15–1.96)**		
Diarrhoeal disease (two-weekly prevalence)	(i) Untreated (ii) Treated (two storage reservoirs) 10^3–10^4 faecal coliforms/100 ml	0–4	(i) 29.0 vs 23.0 (ii) 26.8 vs 23.0	1.33 (0.96–1.85) 1.17 (0.85–1.60)	Farm workers or their children (i) in direct contact with raw wastewater vs not using wastewater for irrigation (rainy season) (ii) in direct contact with wastewater stored in two reservoirs vs not using wastewater for irrigation	Cifuentes (1998)
		5+	(i) 11.8 vs 9.8 (ii) 10.5 vs 9.8	1.10 (0.88–1.38) 1.06 (0.86–1.29)		

Table 3.12 (continued)

Health outcome and outcome measure	Wastewater quality	Age group (years)	Prevalence or incidence of infection (%)	Relative risk or odds ratio (95% confidence interval)	Study group and comparison	Reference
Diarrhoeal disease (weekly prevalence)	Treated (two reservoirs) 10^4 faecal coliforms/100 ml	5–14	(i) 11.0 vs 4.0 (ii) 7.4 vs 3.2	(i) 3.05 (1.67– 5.58)** (ii) 2.34 (1.20– 4.57)*	Children of farm workers with (i) high level of contact with wastewater vs no contact (rainy season) (ii) contact with wastewater vs no contact (dry season)	Blumenthal et al. (2003)

Significance levels: *, $P < 0.05$; **, $P < 0.01$; ***, $P < 0.001$

[a] Crude relative risk calculated from prevalence or incidence data reported.

Table 3.13 Studies of risks to workers and nearby populations: Enteric viruses and bacteria — seroprevalence and seroconversion and relative risks in populations exposed or not exposed to wastewater used for irrigation

Health outcome	Wastewater quality	Age group (years)	Seroprevalence (%) or seroconversion (%)	Relative risk or odds ratio (95% CI)	Study group and comparison	Reference
Echovirus type 4 infection (% seroprevalence and % seroconversion)	Treated Stabilization ponds 5–10 days retention 10^4–10^5 total coliforms/100 ml	(i) 0–5 (ii) 6–17 (iii) 25+	Seroprevalence (i) 83 vs 33 (ii) 73 vs 37 Seroconversion (iii) 63 vs 20	(i) 2.5^a*** (ii) 2.0** (iii) 3.2**	Comparison of rates in kibbutzim population exposed to aerosolized wastewater from kibbutz itself and nearby towns vs kibbutzim not exposed to wastewater (other comparisons given in paper) [Data from 1980 presented; after national outbreak of echovirus 4] No significant differences were found for all other enteroviruses	Fattal et al. (1987)
Poliovirus infection (i) Polio 1 (ii) Polio 2 (iii) Polio 3 (% seroprevalence)	Treated Stabilization ponds 5–10 days retention	<1–60+	(i) 82 vs 86 (ii) 88 vs 91 (iii) 80 vs 82	(i) 0.95^a (ii) 0.97 (iii) 0.98	1980 data shown Comparison of rates in kibbutzim population exposed to aerosolized wastewater from kibbutz itself and nearby towns vs kibbutzim not exposed to wastewater	Margalith, Morag & Fattal (1990)
Legionellosis (% seroprevalence)	Treated Stabilization ponds 5–7 days retention 10^6–10^7 total coliforms/100 ml	18+	4.3 vs 1.4	3.14 (0.89–11.85)[b]	Sewage contact workers vs non-irrigation workers	Fattal et al. (1985)

Table 3.13 (continued)

Health outcome	Wastewater quality	Age group (years)	Seroprevalence (%) or seroconversion (%)	Relative risk or odds ratio (95% CI)	Study group and comparison	Reference
Infection with enteric viruses (seroconversion incidence densities)	Treated Trickling filter effluent 10^6 faecal coliforms/100 ml (1982) Reservoir effluent 10^3–10^4 faecal coliforms/100 ml (1983)	All ages	(i) 5.37 vs 2.55 (ii) 8.34 vs 1.32 (iii) 8.34 vs 5.46 (iv) 8.34 vs 4.68	2.10 (1.56–2.03)[b]*** 6.31 (2.52–15.76)*** 1.56 (0.86–2.84) 1.78 (1.03–3.09)*	(i) Irrigation vs baseline (ii) High exposure: irrigation vs baseline (iii) Irrigation: High aerosol exposure (index >5) vs low (index <1) (iv) Irrigation: High aerosol exposure vs intermediate aerosol exposure (1 ≤ index ≤5)	Camann et al. (1986a)
Rotavirus infection (% seroconversion)	Treated: trickling filter plant, then storage reservoirs	All ages	(i) 1.99 vs 5.34 (ii) 1.54 v 2.50	(i) 0.37 (0.23–0.62)[b]*** (ii) 1.63 (0.70–3.78)[b]	(i) 20 months after start of spray irrigation vs 20 months before irrigation (ii) 10 months spray irrigation with reservoir effluent vs 10 months spray irrigation with trickling filter plant effluent	Ward et al. (1989)
Enteroviruses: coxsackievirus B5 infection (% seroprevalence)	Treated: storage lagoons (over autumn and winter)	Adults	100 vs 52	1.93 (1.36–2.75)[b]*	Comparison of seropositivity in spray irrigation workers vs spray nozzle cleaners No significant differences were found for all other enteroviruses	Linnemann et al. (1984)
Norwalk-like virus: Mexico infection (% seroresponse)	Treated 10^4 faecal coliforms/100 ml	>15	33.3 vs 11.4	4.21 (1.62–10.96)**	Farm workers with high level of contact with wastewater vs no contact	Blumenthal et al. (2003)
Salmonellosis (prevalence)	Untreated	<15	39.3 vs 24.6	1.60**	Children of agriculturalists vs children from non-agricultural families	Ait Melloul & Hassani (1999)

Significance levels: *, $P < 0.05$; **, $P < 0.01$; ***, $P < 0.001$

[a] Crude relative risk calculated from seroprevalence or seroconversion data reported.

[b] Crude relative risk and 95% confidence interval calculated from seroprevalence or seroconversion.

Reported diarrhoeal disease

Analytical studies in Mexico of the effect of direct contact with wastewater indicate that there are risks of diarrhoeal disease related to contact with untreated wastewater, particularly in the dry season (relative risk 1.75), and that the risk is reduced when the wastewater is stored in storage reservoirs before use (Cifuentes, 1998; Blumenthal et al., 2001).

When wastewater was partially treated in a single reservoir (10^5 thermotolerant coliforms per 100 ml) (Blumenthal et al., 2001), there was still an excess risk of diarrhoeal disease in the dry season in children older than five (relative risk 1.5). When it was treated in two reservoirs in series (10^3–10^4 thermotolerant coliforms per 100 ml), no excess risk of diarrhoeal disease was detected in the rainy season (Cifuentes, 1998), unless there were high levels of contact (Blumenthal et al., 2003), but an increased risk was found in school-aged children in the dry season (relative risk 2.3).

Serological studies

In a study in Mexico (Blumenthal et al., 2003), farm workers who had a high level of direct contact with wastewater that had been stored in a single reservoir (quality 10^4 thermotolerant coliforms per 100 ml) had a fourfold increase in seroresponse to norovirus (Mexico strain) infection after allowance for confounding factors.

3.2.3 Risks to local communities from sprinkler irrigation

Table 3.12 summarizes the studies that were reviewed on risks of reported enteric disease to agricultural workers and nearby populations, and Table 3.13 summarizes the serological studies that were reviewed on risks of enteric viruses and bacteria to agricultural workers and nearby populations.

Reported enteric infections

Several studies in Israel have investigated the effect of exposure of the general population to wastewater aerosols from sprinkler irrigation of partially treated wastewater from waste stabilization ponds (short retention times). The most recent study, a prospective cohort study (Shuval et al., 1989), found that episodes of enteric disease were similar in kibbutzim most exposed to treated wastewater aerosols from waste stabilization ponds (10^4–10^5 total coliforms per 100 ml; sprinkler irrigation within 300–600 m of residential areas) and in those not exposed to wastewater in any form. This supersedes the results of the first (Katzenelson, Buiu & Shuval, 1976) and second studies (Fattal et al., 1986), which reported high risks of enteric disease related to exposure to wastewater (10^6–10^8 total coliforms per 100 ml), but which were methodologically flawed.

When effluent from a trickling filter plant in Lubbock in the United States of America was used for irrigation (10^6 thermotolerant coliforms per 100 ml, 100–1000 enteroviruses per 100 ml), there was a borderline association between high aerosol exposure and viral illness ($P = 0.06$), but this disappeared after allowance was made for confounding factors (Camann & Moore, 1987). Exposure to higher-quality wastewater from storage reservoirs (10^3–10^4 thermotolerant coliforms per 100 ml) had no significant effect on viral illness (Moore et al., 1988). Another study in the same country (Linneman et al., 1984) using effluent from storage lagoons (where storage was for about six months) had similar results.

Serological studies of viral and bacterial infections

Serological studies from kibbutzim in Israel (Fattal et al., 1985, 1987; Margalith, Morag & Fattal, 1990) indicate that there is no excess endemic viral infection related to exposure to wastewater aerosols through sprinkler irrigation from 5- to 10-day waste stabilization ponds (wastewater quality 10^6–10^8 total coliforms per 100 ml). There was no significant increase in levels of antibodies to echovirus types 7 and 9, coxsackievirus types A9, B1, B3 and B4 and hepatitis A virus (Fattal et al., 1987) or to poliovirus types 1, 2 and 3 (Margalith, Morag & Fattal, 1990). There was a significant increase in levels of antibodies to echovirus type 4 (but no additional disease incidence), however, in kibbutzim that had been exposed to aerosols of partially treated wastewater from nearby towns (Fattal et al., 1987). This could be attributed to a major epidemic of echovirus 4 in Israel at the time.

In the Lubbock Infection Surveillance Study (Camann et al., 1986a), wastewater irrigation was significantly associated with new viral infections when seroconversion incidence densities for coxsackievirus B and echoviruses were compared before and after irrigation started (Camann et al., 1986a, 1986b), especially in those who had a high degree of aerosol exposure.

Infection episodes ($n = 5$) that were significantly associated with aerosol exposure occurred mainly when effluent from a trickling filter plant (quality 10^6 thermotolerant coliforms per 100 ml, 100–1000 enteroviruses per 100 ml) was being used for irrigation, but not when effluent from storage reservoirs (quality 10^3–10^4 thermotolerant coliforms per 100 ml, <10 enteroviruses per 100 ml) were used. When allowance was made for potential confounding factors, however, the association between exposure and infection was significant ($P < 0.05$) only for two of the five episodes reported (Camann et al., 1986b) where the agents of infection were poliovirus 1 and coxsackievirus B (first episode) and echoviruses (second episode).

In an earlier study (Linneman et al., 1984), no significant differences in seroresponse to infections were found in spray irrigation workers exposed to effluent from storage lagoons except for those who cleaned the nozzles (and were frequently soaked with wastewater), who had higher seroprevalences of coxsackievirus B5.

3.2.4 Overall results for farming families and local communities

There is evidence to suggest that direct contact with untreated wastewater through flood or furrow irrigation can lead to increased helminth infection (mainly *Ascaris* infection) and that this effect is more pronounced in children than in adults. There is some evidence that *Ascaris* infection related to direct contact with wastewater can be reduced when the wastewater is partially treated before use and that the effect depends on the extent of treatment. Treatment may need to achieve concentrations below one egg per litre where children under 15 are exposed, perhaps combined with measures to restrict the contact of children with wastewater through play or work.

Studies of diarrhoeal disease related to direct contact with wastewater suggest that:

- there is an increased risk of diarrhoeal disease, particularly in young children and in the dry season, related to exposure to untreated wastewater;
- partial treatment of the wastewater (to 10^5 thermotolerant coliforms per 100 ml) reduces the effect in adults but not in children;
- treatment may need to be below 10^4 thermotolerant coliforms per 100 ml in circumstances where children have high amounts of contact, or, if this is not possible, effective measures to reduce contact of children with wastewater may need to be introduced.

The better-quality studies of sprinkler irrigation of treated wastewater indicate that there may be an increased risk of infection when the quality of the wastewater is 10^6 thermotolerant coliforms per 100 ml, but no increased risk of infection when the water quality is 10^4–10^5 thermotolerant coliforms per 100 ml or less.

3.3 Quantitative microbial risk analysis

Since the publication of the second edition of these Guidelines in 1989, the development of QMRA has enabled increasingly sophisticated analysis of health risks associated with wastewater use in agriculture. The data generated in these assessments are a useful complement to those available from epidemiological studies. QMRA can estimate risks from a variety of different exposures and/or pathogens that would be difficult to measure through epidemiological investigations due to the high cost and necessity of studying large populations. QMRA has been applied to risks associated with bacteria, protozoa and viruses, but few QMRAs have been conducted on the transmission of helminth infections from wastewater or excreta use activities.

Asano et al. (1992) estimated the risk of infection with three enteric viruses (poliovirus 1 and 3 and echovirus 12) related to use of chlorinated tertiary effluents and unchlorinated secondary effluents given tertiary treatment. Four scenarios of exposure to wastewater were used: (i) irrigation of market garden produce; (ii) irrigation of golf courses; (iii) recreational use of water; and (iv) groundwater recharge. The dose–response model used was the β-Poisson model (Haas, 1983) (see Box 3.1). Asano et al. (1992) used estimates of the amount of water ingested via the various scenarios — for example, 1 ml per day for two days per week throughout the year by golfers handling and cleaning golf balls, and 10 ml per day for consumers of food crops. Allowance was made for viral reduction in the environment — for example, through stopping crop irrigation two weeks before harvest.

The risk of infection related to consuming irrigated "market garden produce" was calculated to be 10^{-6}–10^{-9} per person per year when the effluent contained one viral unit per 100 litres and 10^{-4}–10^{-7} per person per year when the concentration was 111 viral units per 100 litres. The corresponding infection risk estimates were 10^{-11}–10^{-14} per person per year and 10^{-9}–10^{-11} per person per year when unchlorinated secondary effluents with 500 viral units per 100 litres and 73 400 viral units per 100 litres, respectively, were given tertiary treatment (a 5 log unit viral removal). Thus, for all the tertiary effluents investigated, the infection risks were below the accepted infection risk of 10^{-4} per person per year in the United States of America (Rose & Gerba, 1991), and sometimes below this level by many orders of magnitude.

Even when unchlorinated secondary effluents were investigated using viral removal data from wastewater treatment plants in California, USA, QMRA showed that for food crop irrigation and groundwater recharge, the risk of viral infection was less than 10^{-4} per person per year (Tanaka et al., 1998). This study used the same dose–response model as Asano et al. (1992), but used cumulative distribution functions of virus concentrations (instead of point estimates) and 500-trial Monte Carlo simulations. The annual infection risk to consumers from crop irrigation (daily consumption) was calculated for three types of treatment and several treatment plants. The estimates were as follows: 10^{-3}–10^{-5} per person per year for unchlorinated secondary effluent; 10^{-7}–10^{-9} per person per year for direct chlorination of secondary effluent (a 3.9 log unit removal); and 10^{-8}–10^{-10} for full treatment (a 5.2 log unit removal). For golf courses, the annual risks were 10^{-4}–10^{-6} per person per year when

Box 3.1 QMRA: dose–response models

The dose–response models used were the β-Poisson model for rotavirus and *Campylobacter* infections and the exponential model for *Cryptosporidium* infection (Haas et al., 1999). The equations are:

(a) β-Poisson dose–response model (for *Campylobacter* and rotavirus):

$$P_I(d) = 1 - [1 + (d/ID_{50})(2^{1/\alpha} - 1)]^{-\alpha}$$

(b) Exponential dose–response model (for *Cryptosporidium*):

$$P_I(d) = 1 - \exp(-rd)$$

(c) Annual risk of infection:

$$P_{I(A)}(d) = 1 - [1 - P_I(d)]^n$$

where $P_I(d)$ is the risk of infection in an individual exposed to (via ingestion, in this case) a single pathogen dose d; $P_{I(A)}(d)$ is the annual risk of infection in an individual from n exposures per year to the single pathogen dose d; ID_{50} is the median infective dose; and α and r are pathogen "infectivity constants." For rotavirus, $ID_{50} = 6.17$ and $\alpha = 0.253$; for *Campylobacter*, $ID_{50} = 896$ and $\alpha = 0.145$; and for *Cryptosporidium*, $r = 0.0042$ (Haas et al., 1999). $P_{I(A)}(d)$ can also be interpreted as the risk over a shorter (or longer) period — for example, an *m*-month risk, with n now equal to the number of exposures during *m* months.

The value of $P_{I(A)}(d)$ is in the range 0–1. If $P_{I(A)}(d) = 1$, infection is certain. However, QMRA cannot determine whether an individual becomes infected more than once per year. Such information can be found only by epidemiological studies.

chlorinated secondary effluent (a 3.9 log unit removal) was used, but 10^{-1}–10^{-2} per person per year when it was not chlorinated. The estimated risks were higher when treated wastewater was used in recreational impoundments used for swimming.

These studies suggest that (i) using wastewater for crop irrigation may not be as "risky" as using it for the irrigation of golf courses or for recreational impoundments, mainly due to viral reduction in the environment between application and exposure; and (ii) it may be possible to use secondary effluents, especially when they are chlorinated, and still be below the acceptable level of risk to crop consumers.

Shuval, Lampert & Fattal (1997) used QMRA to perform a comparative risk analysis of the USEPA & USAID (1992) guidelines and of the second edition of the WHO Guidelines (WHO, 1989). The risk assessment model developed for studying microorganisms in drinking-water (Haas et al., 1993) was used, combined with laboratory data on the degree of viral contamination of vegetables irrigated with wastewaters of various qualities. They compared estimates of disease risk from the consumption of lettuce (100 g per person on alternate days) that had been irrigated with untreated wastewater and treated wastewater with 10^3 thermotolerant coliforms per 100 ml. The risk of clinical cases of hepatitis A infection from eating lettuce that had been irrigated with untreated wastewater was 10^{-2}–10^{-4} per person per year. However, when the lettuces were irrigated with treated wastewaters containing 10^3 thermotolerant coliforms per 100 ml, the risk was 10^{-6}–10^{-8} per person per year, and the corresponding risk for rotavirus disease was 10^{-5}–10^{-6} per person per year. Fattal, Lampert & Shuval (2004) confirmed these results by a more detailed analysis: the hepatitis A disease risks were 4.4×10^{-2} per person per year when lettuce was irrigated with untreated wastewater and 4.7×10^{-6} per person per year when irrigated with wastewater treated to 10^3 faecal coliforms per 100 ml. The corresponding rotavirus disease risks were 10^{-1} and 10^{-5} per person per year, respectively.

More recently, these pioneering studies by Shuval and colleagues have been extended by D.D. Mara and colleagues (unpublished data, 2005) to provide further information as a basis to evaluate the infection risks. These studies explored exposure through direct contact with wastewater (through restricted irrigation), as well as exposure through crop consumption (through unrestricted irrigation). A combination of standard QMRA techniques (Haas et al., 1999) and 10 000-trial Monte Carlo simulations (Sleigh & Mara, 2003) was used. The risk estimates were determined by using the β-Poisson dose–response model for bacterial and viral infections and the exponential dose–response model for protozoan infections.

The model exposure scenario used for restricted irrigation was the involuntary ingestion of soil particles by those working, or by young children playing, in wastewater-irrigated fields. The quantity of soil involuntarily ingested in this way was up to approximately 100 mg per person per day of exposure (Haas et al., 1999; WHO, 2001b). Two "sub-scenarios" were considered:

- highly mechanized agriculture;
- labour-intensive agriculture.

The first scenario represents exposure in industrialized countries where farm workers typically plough, sow and harvest using tractors and associated equipment and could be expected to wear gloves when working in wastewater-irrigated fields. The second scenario is representative of farming practices in developing countries in situations where tractors are not (or only rarely) used and gloves not commonly worn.

Two exposure scenarios were used for unrestricted irrigation:

- an extended version of the scenario of wastewater-irrigated lettuce consumption used by Shuval, Lampert & Fattal (1997);
- the consumption of uncooked wastewater-irrigated onions, based on the epidemiological study in Mexico detailed by Blumenthal et al. (2003) (section 3.2.1).

These two scenarios were chosen as they cover both root and non-root crops eaten uncooked. The onion consumption scenario permitted a comparison between disease incidences determined epidemiologically and infection risks estimated by QMRA.

For restricted irrigation, D.D. Mara et al. (unpublished data, 2005) estimated the median risks per person per year for rotavirus, *Campylobacter* and *Cryptosporidium* infections resulting from the ingestion of 1–10 mg of wastewater-contaminated soil per person per day for 100 days per year for highly mechanized agriculture and 10–100 mg per person per day for 300 days per year for labour-intensive agriculture. Exposure for 300 days per year was chosen to represent a landless labourer working for two days per week for each of three employers; this exposure represents a "worst-case" scenario, as irrigation does not commonly extend over a full year, although in some cases (e.g. coastal desert areas in South America) it does. The risks were estimated for seven single-log ranges (10–100 to 10^7–10^8) of *E. coli* numbers per 100 ml of wastewater. These log ranges were chosen to estimate the risks associated with different levels of treatment from untreated wastewater through to high-level treatment (e.g. as practised in the State of California, USA) ($\leq$23 total coliforms per 100 ml for restricted irrigation; State of California, 2001), while allowing for any value to be exceeded by up to one order of magnitude.

The estimated infection risks for highly mechanized agriculture, shown in **Table 3.14**, are close to 10^{-3} per person per year for rotavirus infection when the water quality is approximately 10^5 *E. coli* per 100 g of soil. For labour-intensive agriculture with exposure for 300 days per year (**Table 3.15**), the estimated infection risks are close to 10^{-3} per person per year when the water quality is 10^3–10^4 *E. coli* per 100 g of soil. In both scenarios, the risks for *Campylobacter* and *Cryptosporidium* infections were much lower than 10^{-3} per person per year. Table 3.15 also shows that the infection risks resulting from the use of untreated wastewater (10^7–10^8 *E. coli* per 100 g) were substantial: 0.99 per person per year for rotavirus and 0.50 per person per year for *Campylobacter*. When the exposure was for 150 days per year (Table 3.16), the risks were halved.

For unrestricted irrigation, D.D. Mara et al. (unpublished data, 2005) estimated the median risks per person per year for rotavirus, *Campylobacter* and *Cryptosporidium* infections resulting from the consumption of 100 g of wastewater-irrigated lettuce on alternate days. The parameter values used in the models were modified slightly compared with those used by Shuval, Lampert & Fattal (1997) — for example, by extending the die-off of 10^{-3} downwards by one order of magnitude to 10^{-2} and allowing for ±25% of the values of the β-Poisson "infectivity constants" (ID_{50} and α) given in Box 3.1. The risks were estimated for eight single-log ranges (1–10 to 10^7–10^8) of *E. coli* numbers per 100 ml of wastewater. The estimated infection risks, given in Table 3.17, are 10^{-3} per person per year for rotavirus and approximately 10^{-5} per person per year for *Campylobacter* and *Cryptosporidium* for a wastewater quality of 10^3–10^4 *E. coli* per 100 ml (Table 3.17).

D.D. Mara et al. (unpublished data, 2005) also estimated the median risks per person per year for rotavirus, *Campylobacter* and *Cryptosporidium* infections resulting from the consumption of 100 g of raw onions per person per week for five months; these rates of consumption were based on those found in the dry season in the Mezquital Valley in Mexico, where Blumenthal et al. (2003) studied the weekly prevalence of symptomatic diarrhoeal disease. The parameter values used in the models were modified to reflect the field conditions by using different ranges of parameter values, to allow for (a) the greater number of microorganisms expected to be on the surface of onions than on lettuce (Geldreich & Bordner [1971] found root vegetables irrigated with wastewater containing 5.8×10^4 faecal coliforms per 100 ml to have an order-of-magnitude higher count of faecal bacteria than leafy vegetables); (b) the lower die-off of faecal organisms in soil than on exposed crop surfaces (Strauss, 1985); and (c) a lower volume of wastewater remaining on onions than on lettuce.

The simulated rotavirus infection risk of 0.39 per person per five months for a wastewater quality of 10^3–10^5 *E. coli* per 100 ml (Table 3.18) shows very close agreement with the measured incidence of diarrhoeal disease of 0.38 per person per five months (calculated by converting prevalence values obtained in the epidemiological study to estimates of the rate of infection, using a number of assumptions). The risks calculated for *Campylobacter* and *Cryptosporidium* were lower by one and three orders of magnitude, respectively. Thus, provided that the parameter values used in the QMRA equations are carefully chosen to reflect

Table 3.14 Restricted irrigation: highly mechanized agriculture — median infection risks from ingestion of wastewater-contaminated soil estimated by 10 000-trial Monte Carlo simulations[a]

Soil quality (*E. coli* per 100 g)	Median infection risk (per person per year)		
	Rotavirus	*Campylobacter*	*Cryptosporidium*
10^7-10^8	0.50	2.1×10^{-2}	4.7×10^{-4}
10^6-10^7	6.8×10^{-2}	1.9×10^{-3}	4.7×10^{-5}
10^5-10^6	6.7×10^{-3}	1.9×10^{-4}	4.6×10^{-6}
10^4-10^5	6.5×10^{-4}	2.3×10^{-5}	4.6×10^{-7}
10^3-10^4	6.8×10^{-5}	2.4×10^{-6}	5.0×10^{-8}
100–1000	6.3×10^{-6}	2.2×10^{-7}	$\leq 1 \times 10^{-8}$
10–100	6.9×10^{-7}	2.2×10^{-8}	–

[a] 1–10 mg soil ingested per person per day for 100 days per year; 0.1–1 rotavirus and *Campylobacter* and 0.01–0.1 *Cryptosporidium* oocyst per 10^5 *E. coli*; $ID_{50} = 6.17 \pm 25\%$ and $\alpha = 0.253 \pm 25\%$ for rotavirus; $ID_{50} = 896 \pm 25\%$ and $\alpha = 0.145 \pm 25\%$ for *Campylobacter*; $r = 0.0042 \pm 25\%$ for *Cryptosporidium*.

Table 3.15 Restricted irrigation: labour-intensive agriculture with exposure for 300 days per year — median infection risks from ingestion of wastewater-contaminated soil estimated by 10 000-trial Monte Carlo simulations[a]

Soil quality (*E. coli* per 100 g)	Median infection risk (per person per year)		
	Rotavirus	*Campylobacter*	*Cryptosporidium*
10^7-10^8	0.99	0.50	1.4×10^{-2}
10^6-10^7	0.88	6.7×10^{-2}	1.4×10^{-3}
10^5-10^6	0.19	7.3×10^{-3}	1.4×10^{-4}
10^4-10^5	2.0×10^{-2}	7.0×10^{-4}	1.3×10^{-5}
10^3-10^4	1.8×10^{-3}	6.1×10^{-5}	1.4×10^{-6}
100–1000	1.9×10^{-4}	5.6×10^{-6}	1.4×10^{-7}
10–100	2.0×10^{-5}	5.6×10^{-7}	1.4×10^{-8}

[a] 10–100 mg soil ingested per person per day for 300 days per year; 0.1–1 rotavirus and *Campylobacter* and 0.01–0.1 *Cryptosporidium* oocyst per 10^5 *E. coli*; $ID_{50} = 6.17 \pm 25\%$ and $\alpha = 0.253 \pm 25\%$ for rotavirus; $ID_{50} = 896 \pm 25\%$ and $\alpha = 0.145 \pm 25\%$ for *Campylobacter*; $r = 0.0042 \pm 25\%$ for *Cryptosporidium*.

conditions in the field, there can be agreement between QMRA-estimated infection risks and disease incidences determined from epidemiological field studies (this was also found to be the case for restricted wastewater irrigation).

In the approaches discussed above, risks of infection for given wastewater qualities were determined. An alternative approach is to determine wastewater quality, and thus the required level of pathogen reduction in log_{10} units (or percentage removal),[1] for given levels of tolerable infection risks (Table 3.19). This approach is more useful for establishing operational health-based targets (see section 4.2). It has been used in the drafting of Australian guidelines for wastewater use in agriculture (NRMMC & EPHCA, 2005). The starting point of this approach was to set the

---

[1] In these Guidelines, log_{10} unit reductions are generally referred to as log unit reductions. A 1 log unit reduction = 90% reduction; a 2 log unit reduction = 99% reduction; a 3 log unit reduction = 99.9% reduction; and so on.

Table 3.16 Restricted irrigation: labour-intensive agriculture with exposure for 150 days per year — median infection risks from ingestion of wastewater-contaminated soil estimated by 10 000-trial Monte Carlo simulations[a]

Soil quality (E. coli per 100 g)	Median infection risk (per person per year)		
	Rotavirus	Campylobacter	Cryptosporidium
10^7-10^8	0.99	0.29	6.6×10^{-3}
10^6-10^7	0.65	3.1×10^{-2}	6.8×10^{-4}
10^5-10^6	9.9×10^{-2}	3.2×10^{-3}	7.2×10^{-5}
10^4-10^5	9.6×10^{-3}	3.5×10^{-4}	6.8×10^{-6}
10^3-10^4	9.6×10^{-4}	2.9×10^{-5}	7.0×10^{-7}
100–1000	1.1×10^{-4}	3.0×10^{-6}	7.0×10^{-8}
10–100	1.0×10^{-5}	2.9×10^{-7}	7.0×10^{-9}

[a] 10–100 mg soil ingested per person per day for 150 days per year; 0.1–1 rotavirus and *Campylobacter* and 0.01–0.1 *Cryptosporidium* oocyst per 10^5 *E. coli*; $ID_{50} = 6.17 \pm 25\%$ and $\alpha = 0.253 \pm 25\%$ for rotavirus; $ID_{50} = 896 \pm 25\%$ and $\alpha = 0.145 \pm 25\%$ for *Campylobacter*; $r = 0.0042 \pm 25\%$ for *Cryptosporidium*.

Table 3.17 Unrestricted irrigation: median infection risks from the consumption of wastewater-irrigated lettuce estimated by 10 000-trial Monte Carlo simulations[a]

Wastewater quality (E. coli per 100 ml)	Median infection risk (per person per year)		
	Rotavirus	Campylobacter	Cryptosporidium
10^7-10^8	0.99	0.28	0.50
10^6-10^7	0.65	6.3×10^{-2}	6.3×10^{-2}
10^5-10^6	9.7×10^{-2}	2.4×10^{-3}	6.3×10^{-3}
10^4-10^5	9.6×10^{-3}	2.6×10^{-4}	6.8×10^{-4}
10^3-10^4	1.0×10^{-3}	2.6×10^{-5}	3.1×10^{-5}
100–1000	8.6×10^{-5}	3.1×10^{-6}	6.4×10^{-6}
10–100	8.0×10^{-6}	3.1×10^{-7}	6.7×10^{-7}
1–10	1.0×10^{-6}	3.0×10^{-8}	7.0×10^{-8}

[a] 100 g lettuce eaten per person per two days; 10–15 ml wastewater remaining on 100 g lettuce after irrigation; 0.1–1 rotavirus and *Campylobacter* and 0.01–0.1 *Cryptosporidium* oocyst per 10^5 *E. coli*; $10^{-2}-10^{-3}$ rotavirus and *Campylobacter* die-off and 0–0.1 *Cryptosporidium* oocyst die-off between harvest and consumption; $ID_{50} = 6.17 \pm 25\%$ and $\alpha = 0.253 \pm 25\%$ for rotavirus; $ID_{50} = 896 \pm 25\%$ and $\alpha = 0.145 \pm 25\%$ for *Campylobacter*; $r = 0.0042 \pm 25\%$ for *Cryptosporidium*.

tolerable risk at 10^{-6} DALY per person per year and derive the related disease risks for rotavirus, *Campylobacter* and *Cryptosporidium*. These were 2×10^{-3}, 1.3×10^{-4} and 8.7×10^{-4} per person per year, respectively, for an exposure scenario of the irrigation of lettuce consumption, assuming 70 exposure events a year in the Australian context. QMRA was then undertaken to calculate the log unit reduction required to achieve these levels of risk, after inputting data on (i) pathogen concentrations in wastewater, (ii) dose–response data, (iii) exposure per event, (iv) disease/infection ratios, (v) DALYs per case of disease and (vi) susceptibility fractions to account for the proportion of the population who are not immune. The required pathogen reductions were calculated as 5.5 log units for rotavirus, 5 for *Campylobacter* and 4.5 for *Cryptosporidium*. The limitations of this approach included the use of a non–Monte Carlo QMRA model, resulting in the calculation of single point estimates, such that variability and uncertainty were not addressed. The estimates were based on conservative values.

Table 3.18 Unrestricted irrigation: median infection risks from the consumption of wastewater-irrigated onions estimated by 10 000-trial Monte Carlo simulations[a]

Wastewater quality (E. coli per 100 ml)	Median infection risk (per person per year)		
	Rotavirus	*Campylobacter*	*Cryptosporidium*
10^7–10^8	1.00	0.99	3.6×10^{-2}
10^6–10^7	0.99	0.81	3.9×10^{-3}
10^5–10^6	0.99	0.17	3.2×10^{-4}
10^4–10^5	0.43	1.6×10^{-2}	3.7×10^{-5}
10^3–10^5	0.39	1.7×10^{-2}	2.8×10^{-4}
3×10^4	0.29	1.1×10^{-2}	2.3×10^{-4}
10^3–10^4	4.5×10^{-2}	2.6×10^{-5}	3.7×10^{-6}
100–1000	5.6×10^{-3}	1.0×10^{-4}	3.8×10^{-7}
10–100	4.4×10^{-4}	1.1×10^{-5}	3.0×10^{-8}
1–10	5.7×10^{-5}	1.8×10^{-6}	$<10^{-8}$

[a] 100 g of onions consumed per person once per week for five months; 1–5 ml wastewater remaining on 100 g onions after irrigation; 1–10 rotavirus and *Campylobacter* and 0.1–1 *Cryptosporidium* oocyst per 10^5 *E. coli*; 0.1–1 rotavirus and *Campylobacter* die-off and 0.01–0.1 *Cryptosporidium* oocyst die-off between harvest and consumption; $ID_{50} = 6.17 \pm 25\%$ and $\alpha = 0.253 \pm 25\%$ for rotavirus; $ID_{50} = 896 \pm 25\%$ and $\alpha = 0.145 \pm 25\%$ for *Campylobacter*; $r = 0.0042 \pm 25\%$ for *Cryptosporidium*.

3.4 Emerging issues: infectious diseases

One study has demonstrated that *E. coli* O157:H7 could be taken into lettuce plants and seedlings from contaminated irrigation water and manure slurries systemically through the roots, resulting in contamination of the edible parts of the plant (Solomon, Yaron & Matthews, 2002). If more evidence for this type of pathogen uptake is discovered, this would have important implications for the use of manure slurries (and, to a lesser extent, wastewater) for the production of vegetables that are consumed raw. *E. coli* O157:H7 is of particular concern because of its ability to survive in the environment (Wang, Zhao & Doyle, 1996), its relatively low infectious dose ($<10^3$ bacteria) (Ackers et al., 1998) and its potential for causing severe health outcomes in susceptible populations (e.g. children, the elderly and the immunocompromised). Studies from the United States of America detected *E. coli* O157:H7 in one of six samples (approximately 17%) of raw wastewater (Grant et al., 1996). In South Africa, similar results were found in a larger set of wastewater samples (16/91 samples; 17.6%) (Müller, Grabow & Ehlers, 2003). More research is needed to find out how widespread this phenomenon is and its public health significance.

3.5 Chemicals

Toxic chemicals are a growing concern in some regions. The number of toxic chemicals used in households and industry is large and growing. This section examines the health issues associated with toxic chemicals that have been found in wastewater. In general, industrial wastewater discharges into sanitary sewers or drains are the source of many chemicals, although households may also contribute. By limiting toxic chemical discharges into municipal wastewater, the hazard to public health and the environment can be reduced. A risk analysis was carried out to determine which chemicals potentially pose the greatest risks to human health. Section 4.6 gives health-based maximum soil concentrations for certain chemicals to prevent their entrance into the food-chain.

Table 3.19 Unrestricted irrigation: required pathogen reductions for various levels of tolerable risk of infection from the consumption of wastewater-irrigated lettuce and onions estimated by 10 000-trial Monte Carlo simulations[a]

Tolerable level of infection risk (per person per year)	Corresponding required level of reduction (log units)	
	Lettuce	Onions
Rotavirus		
10^{-2}	5	6
10^{-3}	6	7
10^{-4}	7	8
Campylobacter		
10^{-2}	4	4
10^{-3}	5	5
10^{-4}	6	6
Cryptosporidium		
10^{-2}	4	2
10^{-3}	5	3
10^{-4}	6	4

[a] 100 g lettuce and onions eaten per person per two days; 10–15 ml and 1–5 ml wastewater remaining after irrigation on 100 g lettuce and 100 g onions, respectively; 0.1–1 and 1–5 rotavirus and *Campylobacter* and 0.1–1 *Cryptosporidium* oocyst per 10^5 *E. coli* for lettuce and onions, respectively; $ID_{50} = 6.17 \pm 25\%$ and $\alpha = 0.253 \pm 25\%$ for rotavirus; $ID_{50} = 896 \pm 25\%$ and $\alpha = 0.145 \pm 25\%$ for *Campylobacter*; $r = 0.0042 \pm 25\%$ for *Cryptosporidium*.

Industrial and, to a lesser extent, municipal wastewaters are sources of chemical pollutants that may affect human health. Tens of thousands of chemicals are used routinely in manufacturing, agricultural production and household products. A fraction of these potentially toxic chemicals may find their way into wastewater collection systems. Chemical contaminants of potential health concern that have been found in wastewater are shown in Table 4.7 in chapter 4.

The health risks associated with chemicals found in wastewater may need to be given more attention, particularly in developing countries where the pace of industrialization is accelerating and where industrial discharges and municipal wastewater are frequently mixed together.

3.5.1 Health impacts
Direct health impacts

Evidence for direct health impacts from chemical exposures associated with the use of wastewater in agriculture is very limited. This is probably due to the nature of chemical toxicity. For most chemicals, their concentrations in wastewater or wastewater-irrigated products will almost never be high enough to result in acute health effects. Chronic health effects that may be associated with exposure to chemicals in wastewater (e.g. cancer) usually occur only after many years of exposure and may also result from a variety of other exposures not related to the agricultural use of wastewater.

Nevertheless, health effects associated with the use of water heavily contaminated with industrial discharges have been reported. In Japan, Itai-itai disease, a bone and kidney disorder associated with chronic cadmium poisoning, occurred in areas where rice paddies were irrigated with water from the contaminated Jinzu River (WHO,

1992). In some parts of China, the use of industrial wastewater for irrigation was associated with a 36% increase in hepatomegaly (enlarged liver) and a 100% increase in both cancer and congenital malformation rates (Yuan, 1993).

Indirect health impacts

Poor irrigation practices with untreated or partially treated wastewater also impact the quality and safety of groundwater in shallow aquifers and surface waters that may supply drinking-water. Wastewater-related nitrate contamination of aquifers has been extensively documented in both developed and developing countries. High concentrations of nitrate in drinking-water are associated with methaemoglobinaemia ("blue baby" syndrome). Some cases of methaemoglobinaemia associated with nitrate exposure in bottle-fed infants have been reported in Eastern Europe and the United States of America, including several infant deaths (Knobeloch et al., 2000; WHO, 2004a).

Excessive nutrients, primarily nitrogen and phosphorus, in wastewater may contaminate surface waters and can cause eutrophication (nutrient enrichment). Eutrophication of fresh water and salt water may create environmental conditions that favour the growth of toxin-producing cyanobacteria and algae. The resulting toxins can cause gastroenteritis, liver damage, nervous system impairment and skin irritation. Health problems associated with cyanotoxins have been documented in several countries, including Australia, Brazil, Canada, China, the United Kingdom, the United States of America and Zimbabwe. In some cases, liver cancer in humans is thought to be associated with exposure to cyanobacterial toxins (microcystins) through drinking-water (Ling, 2000). Exposure to these toxins has usually been through contaminated drinking-water or recreational water contact (Chorus & Bartram, 1999).

3.5.2 Assessing the risks from chemical contaminants

The use of wastewater may introduce potentially toxic pollutants into soils. Through food-chain transfer, toxic pollutants may affect the health and well-being of consumers, as plants absorb the chemicals from the soils. Pollutants accumulated in the soil as the result of wastewater irrigation may subsequently contaminate surface water and groundwater, resulting in additional exposures.

Based on surveys conducted in many parts of the world, certain chemical constituents, such as heavy metals, appear to be ubiquitous and can be found in almost any municipal wastewater stream; others, especially organic chemicals, are present only in some wastewaters or are present only sometimes (WHO, 1975; USEPA, 1990). The presence of a chemical in one wastewater stream is no indicator for its presence or absence in another wastewater stream.

Based on a review of the literature, Chang et al. (2002) identified several inorganic elements and organic compounds that might pose health risks through the use of wastewater (and sludge) in agriculture (see Table 4.7 in chapter 4). These chemicals were identified as having the following properties:

- They are known to be toxic to humans or animals.
- They have been found in wastewaters and/or sewage sludge.
- They may be readily absorbed from soils by plants.

Inorganic elements

Plant uptake of heavy metals is highly dependent on soil conditions, including pH, the presence of other heavy metals, organic matter content, the application of chemical fertilizers, liming, ploughing and water management (Chen, 1992). These factors greatly influence the bioavailability of specific heavy metals. Alloway & Morgan (1986) found that nickel applied to soil in organic substrates (e.g. sewage sludge) was taken up more readily by plants than when the nickel was introduced in an inorganic substrate. Plants absorb more cadmium and lead from acidic soils than from neutral soils (Chen, Lee & Liu, 1997). In some cases, the presence or absence of other divalent metals in the soil can influence the uptake of heavy metals; for example, calcium, zinc and manganese are thought to compete with cadmium for uptake by plants (Cox, 2000).

All of the inorganic elements in Table 4.7 (in chapter 4) occur naturally in soils. Many of them are biologically beneficial in small quantities and will become harmful only at high levels of exposure. For some inorganic elements (e.g. cobalt and copper), no toxicological threshold has been established; for others (e.g. boron, fluorine and zinc), the thresholds are relatively high. Cobalt, copper and zinc are not likely to be absorbed by plants in sufficient quantities to be harmful to consumers. A toxicological threshold has been established for chromate ion (Cr^{6+}). Chromate is rapidly reduced to Cr^{3+}, however, which forms a less soluble solid phase in wastewater or soils. For these reasons, cobalt, copper, zinc and chromium may be ignored (and are not included in Table 4.7).

The inclusion of molybdenum and especially boron in this list is debatable, because boric acid is a commonly used household chemical and has not been associated with human toxicity (it is, however, toxic to some plants; see Annex 1). Molybdenum is considered to be an essential element. Studies on its toxicity to humans through drinking-water exposures have indicated a no-observed-adverse-effect level (NOAEL) of 0.2 mg/l (WHO, 2004a); however, it is unclear if this finding could be extrapolated to food products. The tolerable daily intake (TDI) for boron is estimated to be 0.16 mg/kg of body weight (WHO, 2004a). The oral reference doses established for these chemicals were derived from limited animal bioassay data (WHO, 2004a). Boron, molybdenum and fluorine form anions in soils and, under appropriate circumstances, may be readily absorbed by plants and thus enter the human food-chain.

Organic chemicals
Many of the organic chemicals in Table 4.7 are industrial solvents and are expected to be removed or degraded during wastewater treatment or sludge digestion. Results of the national sewage sludge survey conducted by the USEPA (1990) indicated that the frequency of detection for the majority of these organic chemicals was less than 10%. When they were found in sewage sludge, their concentrations were low. They probably do not need to be considered in wastewater use in agriculture. However, since raw and poorly treated wastewaters are frequently used for crop irrigation in some regions of the world, these chemicals should be included in the assessment. The potential impact of these chemicals on human health needs to be quantified in any toxicity assessment.

3.5.3 Emerging issues: chemicals
Chemicals that mimic hormones or have antihormonal activity, and so interfere with the functioning of endocrine systems in various species, have been identified in municipal wastewaters. Endocrine disruptors, as they are known, derive from many sources, including pesticides, persistent organic pollutants, non-ionic detergents and human and veterinary pharmaceutical residues. Many of these substances are resistant

to conventional wastewater treatment and may persist in the environment for some time (National Research Council, 1998). Human health effects potentially linked to exposure to these chemicals include breast, prostate and testicular cancers, diminished semen quantity and quality and impaired behavioural/mental, immune and thyroid functions in children. Although direct evidence of adverse health effects in humans is lacking, reproductive abnormalities, altered immune function and population disruption potentially linked to exposure to these substances have been observed in amphibians, birds, fish, invertebrates, reptiles and mammals (IPCS, 2002).

Many of the organic compounds identified through the hazard identification process and included in Table 4.7 exhibit endocrine-disrupting characteristics. They are the halogenated organic chemicals (aldrin and dieldrin), plasticizers (phthalates), polycyclic aromatic hydrocarbons (PAHs; e.g. benzo[*a*]pyrene and pyrene), polychlorinated biphenyls (PCBs) and dioxins. Further studies are needed on these substances to assess the potential health and environmental risks they pose during the use of wastewater for crop irrigation.

Pharmaceutically active chemical substances are ubiquitous in municipal wastewater and its treatment by-products. They are released to the terrestrial environment when the wastewater and sewage sludge are applied on cropland or discharged into a receiving water body (Barnes et al., 2002). It appears, from the limited data in the literature, that the compounds are strongly adsorbed by soil organic matter, and they are therefore unlikely to accumulate in the harvested plants (see chapter 7) to levels that, when consumed, would constitute a health risk. No adverse health effects in humans from exposure to these chemicals resulting from wastewater use in agriculture have been documented.

4
HEALTH-BASED TARGETS

This chapter describes the derivation of health-based targets based on a reference or tolerable level of health risk, as described in section 2.4. To achieve the health-based targets, microbial reduction targets are developed. These are described for different irrigation scenarios (i.e. unrestricted, restricted and localized). Parameters to be monitored for verification of microbial reduction targets and other health protection measures are also presented. Countries will be able to use the information in this chapter to develop their own standards. In some cases, the development of different standards for food for export and for food for local consumption will be warranted. Issues surrounding standards for food exports and local consumption are described in sections 4.4 and 4.5. Section 4.6 presents health-based targets that have been derived for selected toxic chemicals.

4.1 Tolerable burden of disease and health-based targets

The most appropriate metric for expressing the burden of a disease is the DALY (Murray & Acharya, 1997) (see Box 2.1 in chapter 2). WHO (2004a) has adopted, in the third edition of the *Guidelines for drinking-water quality*, a tolerable burden of waterborne disease from consuming drinking-water of $\leq 10^{-6}$ DALY per person per year. This value corresponds to a tolerable excess lifetime risk of fatal cancer of 10^{-5} per person (i.e. an individual has a 1 in 100 000 lifetime chance of developing fatal cancer) from consuming drinking-water containing a carcinogen at its guideline value concentration in drinking-water (WHO, 2004a). This level of disease burden can be compared with a mild but more frequent illness such as self-limiting diarrhoea caused by a microbial pathogen. The estimated disease burden associated with mild diarrhoea (e.g. with a case fatality rate of approximately 1×10^{-5}) at an annual disease risk of 1 in 1000 (10^{-3}) (approximately 1 in 10 lifetime risk) is also about 1×10^{-6} DALY (1 µDALY) per person per year (WHO, 2004a). Such a high level of health protection is required for drinking-water, since it is expected to be "safe" by those who drink it. Since food crops irrigated with treated wastewater, especially those eaten uncooked, are also expected to be as safe as drinking-water by those who eat them, the same high health protection level of $\leq 10^{-6}$ DALY per person per year is used for wastewater use in agriculture (see Table 4.1).

Thus, the health-based target adopted in this edition of these Guidelines is a tolerable additional disease burden of $\leq 10^{-6}$ DALY per person per year. For operational purposes, it is also necessary to calculate the corresponding degree of pathogen reduction that achieves this level of health protection and to define appropriate verification measures. This can be done by following the step-by-step approach outlined below.

4.1.1 Step 1: Tolerable risk of infection

"Translate" the tolerable additional annual burden of disease into the equivalent tolerable annual risks of infection and disease due to the pathogen of concern (e.g. *Campylobacter*, *Cryptosporidium*, rotavirus), as follows (where pppy = per person per year):

$$\text{Tolerable disease risk pppy} = \frac{\text{Tolerable DALYs pppy}}{\text{DALYs per case of disease}}$$

Table 4.2 gives the population-based estimates for the DALYs per case of rotavirus disease, campylobacteriosis and cryptosporidiosis (including mortality and, for campylobacteriosis, morbidity due to reactive arthritis and Guillain-Barré syndrome) and the calculated tolerable disease risks.

59

Table 4.1 Health-based targets for treated wastewater use in agriculture

Exposure scenario	Health-based target (DALY per person per year)	Log$_{10}$ pathogen reduction needed[a]	Number of helminth eggs per litre
Unrestricted irrigation	≤10^{-6} [a]		
Lettuce		6	≤1[b,c]
Onion		7	≤1[b,c]
Restricted irrigation	≤10^{-6} [a]		
Highly mechanized		3	≤1[b,c]
Labour intensive		4	≤1[b,c]
Localized (drip) irrigation	≤10^{-6} [a]		
High-growing crops		2	No recommendation[d,e]
Low-growing crops		4	≤1[c,d]

[a] Rotavirus reduction. The health-based target can be achieved, for unrestricted and localized irrigation, by a 6–7 log unit pathogen reduction (obtained by a combination of wastewater treatment and other health protection measures, including an estimated 3–4 log unit pathogen reduction as a result of the natural die-off rate of pathogens under field conditions and the removal of pathogens from irrigated crops by normal domestic washing and rinsing; see section 4.2.1 for further details); for restricted irrigation, it is achieved by a 2–3 log unit pathogen reduction (section 4.2.2).

[b] When children under 15 are exposed, additional health protection measures should be used (e.g. treatment to ≤0.1 egg per litre, protective equipment such as gloves or shoes/boots or chemotherapy; see sections 4.2.1 and 4.2.2 for details).

[c] An arithmetic mean should be determined throughout the irrigation season. The mean value of ≤1 egg per litre should be obtained for at least 90% of samples in order to allow for the occasional high-value sample (i.e. with >10 eggs per litre). With some wastewater treatment processes (e.g. waste stabilization ponds), the hydraulic retention time can be used as a surrogate to assure compliance with ≤1 egg per litre, as explained in section 5.6.1 and Box 5.2.

[d] See section 4.2.3.

[e] No crops to be picked up from the soil.

The tolerable disease risks are in the range 10^{-3}–10^{-4} per person per year and are conservative values, given that the current global incidence of diarrhoeal disease in the age group 5–80+ is in the range 0.1–1 per person per year (see Table 2.4 in chapter 2).

If there are reliable epidemiological data available that show that these risks of disease are not exceeded by a given combination of health-based protection measures (see Table 4.3 below), it is not necessary to undertake steps 2–4 below, and all that remains to be done in such cases is to establish the treatment verification monitoring level (step 5).

The tolerable disease risks are now converted into a tolerable infection risk per person per year by knowing (or making a reasonable assumption about) the proportion of those infected who become ill — the disease/infection ratio. Table 4.2 gives the values for the disease/infection ratios and the resulting tolerable infection risks for these three diseases. Thus, a "design" value of the tolerable infection risk for rotavirus of 10^{-3} per person per year is adopted (see section 4.2).

Table 4.2 DALYs, disease risks, disease/infection ratios and tolerable infection risks for rotavirus, *Campylobacter* and *Cryptosporidium*

Pathogen	DALYs per case of disease[a]	Disease risk pppy equivalent to 10^{-6} DALY pppy	Disease/ infection ratio	Tolerable infection risk pppy[b]
Rotavirus:				
(1) IC	1.4×10^{-2}	7.1×10^{-5}	0.05^{c}	1.4×10^{-3}
(2) DC	$2.6 \times 10^{-2\,c}$	3.8×10^{-5}	0.05^{c}	7.7×10^{-4}
Campylobacter	4.6×10^{-3}	2.2×10^{-4}	0.7	3.1×10^{-4}
Cryptosporidium	1.5×10^{-3}	6.7×10^{-4}	0.3	2.2×10^{-3}

IC, industrialized countries; DC, developing countries; pppy, per person per year
[a] Values from Havelaar & Melse (2003).
[b] Tolerable infection risk = disease risk ÷ disease/infection ratio.
[c] For developing counties, the DALYs per rotavirus death have been reduced by 95%, as approximately 95% of these deaths occur in children under the age of two who are not exposed to wastewater-irrigated foods. The disease/infection ratio for rotavirus is low, as immunity is mostly developed by the age of three.

4.1.2 Step 2: QMRA
Determine, by QMRA, the corresponding pathogen reduction that needs to be achieved. The first step is to determine the maximum number of pathogens ingested per exposure event (e.g. for unrestricted irrigation, the maximum tolerable number of pathogens remaining on the surface of the crop, usually a salad crop [such as lettuce] or a vegetable that may be eaten uncooked [such as cabbage, carrots], at the time of consumption).

4.1.3 Step 3: Required pathogen reduction
Knowing (or estimating) the volume of treated wastewater remaining on the crop following final irrigation (ml of wastewater per 100 g crop), determine the required degree of pathogen reduction to achieve the tolerable additional disease burden of $\leq 10^{-6}$ DALY per person per year. This step requires the numbers of pathogens present in the untreated wastewater to be known or estimated (e.g. in the QMRA calculations in section 3.3 it was assumed that there were 0.01–1 rotavirus and *Campylobacter* and 0.01–0.1 *Cryptosporidium* oocysts per 10^5 *E. coli*).

4.1.4 Step 4: Health-based protection measures to achieve required pathogen reduction
Specify how this pathogen reduction is to be achieved. It can be achieved by wastewater treatment alone or, more commonly, by wastewater treatment in conjunction with other health protection measures, as explained in Table 4.3 and section 4.2 below.

4.1.5 Step 5: Verification monitoring
For viral and bacterial infections, establish the treatment verification monitoring level in terms of *E. coli* (or thermotolerant coliforms) numbers in the final effluent of the wastewater treatment plant, as shown in Table 4.5 below. For helminth infections, establish the treatment verification monitoring level in terms of number of helminth eggs per litre, as shown in Table 4.4 below.

4.1.6 Example derivation of microbial performance targets
Box 4.1 illustrates how this process can be used to derive microbial performance targets for unrestricted irrigation.

Box 4.1 Derivation of microbial performance targets for unrestricted irrigation

This example illustrates how the five-step procedure developed in section 4.1 may be used to derive a health-based operational target for unrestricted crop irrigation with treated wastewater. The parameter values used in steps 2–4 have been chosen solely for the purpose of illustrating this procedure.

Step 1: Tolerable risk of infection
As explained in section 4.1, the "design" risk of rotavirus infection is 10^{-3} per person per year.

Step 2: QMRA
Consumer exposure to pathogens is calculated by using the following illustrative parameter values in the QMRA:

- 5000 rotaviruses per litre of untreated wastewater;
- 10 ml of treated wastewater remaining on 100 g lettuce after irrigation;
- 100 g lettuce consumed per person every second day throughout the year.

The rotavirus dose per exposure (d) is the number of rotaviruses on 100 g lettuce at the time of consumption. The dose is determined by QMRA, for which the equations are (Haas et al., 1999):

(a) Conversion of the tolerable infection risk of 10^{-3} per person per year to the risk of infection per person per exposure event (i.e. per consumption of 100 g lettuce, which takes place every two days throughout the year) [$P_I(d)$]:

$$P_I(d) = 1 - (1 - 10^{-3})^{[1/(365/2)]} = 5.5 \times 10^{-6}$$

(b) Calculation of the dose per exposure event from the β-Poisson dose–response equation:

$$P_I(d) = 1 - [1 + (d/N_{50})(2^{1/\alpha} - 1)]^{-\alpha}$$

i.e.:

$$d = \{[1 - P_I(d)]^{-1/\alpha} - 1\}/\{N_{50}/(2^{1/\alpha} - 1)\}$$

where the values of the dimensionless "infectivity constants" for rotavirus are $N_{50} = 6.17$ and $\alpha = 0.253$.

Thus:

$$d = \{[1 - (5.5 \times 10^{-6})]^{-1/0.253} - 1\}/\{6.17/(2^{1/0.253} - 1)\} = 5 \times 10^{-5} \text{ per exposure event}$$

Step 3: Required pathogen reduction
This dose of 5×10^{-5} rotavirus is contained in the 10 ml remaining on the lettuce at the time of consumption — i.e. a rotavirus concentration of 5×10^{-3} per litre. The number of rotaviruses in the raw wastewater is 5000 per litre, and therefore the required pathogen reduction in $\log_{10}$ units is:

$$\log_{10}(5000) - \log_{10}(5 \times 10^{-3}) = 3.7 - (-2.3) = 6$$

Box 4.1 (continued)

Step 4: Health-based protection measures to achieve required pathogen reduction
The required rotavirus reduction is 6 log units. In this example, it is assumed that there is a 2 log unit pathogen reduction between last irrigation and consumption (due to a combination of, for example, 1 log unit due to pathogen die-off and 1 log unit due to produce washing; see Table 4.3 below). Taking this 2 log unit reduction into account, the wastewater treatment plant has to achieve a 4 log unit pathogen reduction — i.e. a reduction of rotavirus numbers from 5000 per litre in the raw wastewater to 0.5 per litre in the treated wastewater.

Step 5: Verification monitoring
This 4 log unit pathogen reduction by treatment is verified not by measuring pathogen numbers in samples of raw wastewater and treatment plant effluent, but by the reduction in numbers of a pathogen indicator organism. *Escherichia coli* is recommended for this purpose, although thermotolerant coliforms may be used instead. Table 4.5 below gives *E. coli* verification numbers per 100 ml for various required reductions of viral, bacterial and protozoan pathogens (Table 4.4 below gives helminth egg verification numbers per litre for various required reductions of helminth eggs). In this example, an *E. coli* verification level of $\leq 10^3$ would be adopted for monitoring purposes.

4.2 Microbial reduction targets

The approach adopted in these Guidelines focuses on risks from the consumption of food crops eaten uncooked and risks to fieldworkers from direct contact with treated wastewater, for unrestricted and restricted wastewater irrigation, respectively. Data on the health effects of using wastewater in agriculture, including data from epidemiological, microbiological and QMRA studies, were used to assess the infectious disease risks from the use of treated and partially treated wastewater in agriculture. Analysis of the risks resulting from exposure to wastewaters of different qualities was performed. Data developed through Monte Carlo–based QMRA and epidemiological studies (with verification of the Monte Carlo–QMRA models) supported the process of deriving health-based targets directly from these data. Monte Carlo–QMRA was used to generate estimates of infection over a wider range of wastewater qualities, as described in section 3.3. The analyses took account of consumption of crops eaten raw and of risks from direct contact with wastewater (involving involuntary soil ingestion), so that performance targets could be derived for restricted irrigation (where the exposure of farm workers and their children is the exposure of concern), as well as for unrestricted irrigation. The results of these analyses were then checked against the results obtained from relevant epidemiological studies.

4.2.1 Unrestricted irrigation
Microbial reduction targets for viral, bacterial and protozoan pathogens
The Monte Carlo–QMRA results for unrestricted irrigation, based on the exposure scenario of lettuce consumption (section 3.3), together with the relevant epidemiological evidence (section 3.2), show that, in order to achieve $\leq 10^{-6}$ DALY per person per year for rotavirus, a total pathogen reduction of 6 log units for the consumption of leaf crops (lettuce) and 7 log units for the consumption of root crops (onions) is required (see Table 3.19 in chapter 3). In these Guidelines, a pathogen reduction of 6–7 log units is used as the performance target for unrestricted irrigation to achieve the tolerable additional disease burden of $\leq 10^{-6}$ DALY per person per year. Because the risks associated with exposure to rotavirus are estimated to be the highest, this level of pathogen reduction will provide sufficient protection against bacterial and protozoal infections.

A 6–7 log unit pathogen reduction may be achieved by the application of appropriate health protection measures, each of which has its own associated log unit reduction or range of reductions (Table 4.3). A combination of these measures is used such that, for all combinations, the sum of the individual log unit reductions for each health protection measure adopted is equal to the required overall reduction of 6–7 log units.

Table 4.3 Pathogen reductions achievable by various health protection measures

Control measure[a]	Pathogen reduction (log units)	Notes
Wastewater treatment	1–6	The required pathogen reduction to be achieved by wastewater treatment depends on the combination of health protection measures selected (as illustrated in Figure 4.1; pathogen reductions for different wastewater treatment options are presented in chapter 5).
Localized (drip) irrigation (low-growing crops)	2	Root crops and crops such as lettuce that grow just above, but partially in contact with, the soil
Localized (drip) irrigation (high-growing crops)	4	Crops, such as tomatoes, the harvested parts of which are not in contact with the soil
Spray drift control (spray irrigation)	1	Use of micro-sprinklers, anemometer-controlled direction-switching sprinklers, inward-throwing sprinklers, etc.
Spray buffer zone (spray irrigation)	1	Protection of residents near spray or sprinkler irrigation. The buffer zone should be 50–100 m.
Pathogen die-off	0.5–2 per day	Die-off on crop surfaces that occurs between last irrigation and consumption. The log unit reduction achieved depends on climate (temperature, sunlight intensity, humidity), time, crop type, etc.
Produce washing with water	1	Washing salad crops, vegetables and fruit with clean water
Produce disinfection	2	Washing salad crops, vegetables and fruit with a weak disinfectant solution and rinsing with clean water
Produce peeling	2	Fruits, root crops
Produce cooking	6–7	Immersion in boiling or close-to-boiling water until the food is cooked ensures pathogen destruction.

Sources: Beuchat (1998); Petterson & Ashbolt (2003); NRMMC & EPHCA (2005).
[a] These are described in detail in chapter 5.

Figure 4.1 shows pathogen reductions achieved by several options for combining wastewater treatment and other health protection measures to achieve $\leq 10^{-6}$ DALY per person per year. The options in Figure 4.1 represent examples of combinations of health protection measures that can achieve the health-based target in practice. Other combinations are also possible. Planners and designers of wastewater use schemes may wish to explore and/or use a variety of health protection measure combinations that are locally feasible to implement. New treatment technologies may also offer the opportunity of developing new options.

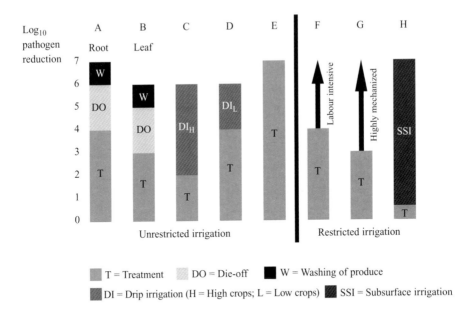

Figure 4.1
Examples of options for the reduction of viral, bacterial and protozoan pathogens by different combinations of health protection measures that achieve the health-based target of $\leq 10^{-6}$ DALY per person per year

Option A in Figure 4.1 shows that the required pathogen reduction is achieved by the combination of (a) wastewater treatment, which provides a 4 log unit pathogen reduction, (b) pathogen die-off between the last irrigation and consumption (a 2 log unit reduction) and (c) washing the salad crops or vegetables with water prior to consumption (a 1 log unit reduction). This option, which provides a 7 log unit pathogen reduction, is suitable when root crops that may be eaten uncooked are irrigated with treated wastewater. This is similar to a recommended required effluent quality of 1000 thermotolerant coli/100 ml in the second edition of these guidelines (WHO, 1989).

Option B has a lower degree of wastewater treatment than Option A (3 log units, rather than 4) combined with two post-treatment health protection measures: a 2 log unit reduction due to die-off and a 1 log unit reduction due to washing the salad crops or vegetables with water prior to consumption. This option, which provides a 6 log unit pathogen reduction, is suitable for the irrigation of non-root salad crops and vegetables eaten uncooked. This provides a sufficient level of health protection because salad crops often have less contamination than root crops and thus consuming them poses less health risk (see Tables 3.17 and 3.18 in chapter 3). This is similar to the recommended required effluent quality of 10,000 thermotolerant coli/100 ml in the second edition of these guidelines (WHO,1989).

Option C combines an even lower degree of treatment (2 log units) but with drip irrigation of high-growing crops (such as tomatoes), which achieves the required remaining 4 log unit pathogen reduction.

Option D incorporates the drip irrigation of low-growing non-root crops (a 2 log unit reduction), so a greater degree of treatment (4 log units) is provided (a valid alternative would be, for example, a 2 log unit reduction by treatment followed by a 1 log unit reduction due to die-off and a 1 log unit reduction due to produce washing).

Option E relies solely on wastewater treatment to achieve the required 6–7 log unit reduction. A typical sequence of wastewater treatment processes to achieve this would comprise conventional wastewater treatment (e.g. primary sedimentation, activated sludge, including secondary sedimentation) followed by chemical coagulation, flocculation, sedimentation and disinfection (chlorination or ultraviolet irradiation). Such a sequence is used, for example, in California, USA, to ensure compliance with the state water recycling criteria for unrestricted irrigation (≤2.2 total coliforms per 100 ml and a turbidity of ≤2 nephelometric turbidity units) (State of California, 2001). This option does not take into account pathogen reduction due to (a) natural die-off between final irrigation and consumption and (b) specific food preparation practices at the household level, such as washing, disinfection, peeling and/or cooking, and overall health protection is therefore greater than even 10^{-6} DALY per person per year. The very high costs and operational complexity of the wastewater treatment processes required for this option will generally preclude its application in many countries. Even in countries where this option is affordable, it should be subject to a robust cost-effectiveness analysis.

Options F, G and H in Figure 4.1 relate to restricted irrigation and are discussed in section 4.2.2. The in-depth risk analyses carried out by scientific communitity working on safe use of wastewater provide the basis for these recommended options. They take into account ecology, epidemiology, human behaviour and cost-effectiveness.

Microbial reduction targets for helminth eggs

Microbial reduction targets for protection against helminth infections are based on the results of epidemiological and microbiological studies. QMRA was not used to derive these performance targets, as there are no credible data on the infection risks and DALYs per person per year resulting from wastewater-related exposures or the infectivity constants for relevant helminths, such as *Ascaris*, for use in QMRA calculations. Furthermore, it is the intensity of the infection, rather than simply infection, that is associated with disability resulting from helminth infections.

Epidemiological studies of *Ascaris* infection among consumers (section 3.2.1) have indicated that wastewater treatment reduces the risk of *Ascaris* infection to adult consumers of crops irrigated with raw wastewater. The value of ≤1 helminth egg per litre is supported by microbiological evidence from field studies in Brazil (section 3.1.1) that, when facultative pond effluent with <0.5 egg per litre was used for irrigation, no eggs were detected on the crops. Therefore, a performance target of ≤1 helminth egg per litre of treated wastewater is recommended for unrestricted irrigation.

Epidemiological studies in Central Mexico (section 3.2.1) indicate that the achievement of ≤1 egg per litre may not be sufficiently protective in situations where conditions favour egg survival (e.g. warm, moist soil conditions), thus allowing for accumulation of eggs on the soil or on the crops, especially where children under the age of 15 consume uncooked food crops brought home from the field by their fieldworker parents. Thus, when children under 15 are exposed by eating uncooked field vegetables (as opposed to commercial food crops) that have been irrigated with treated wastewaters containing ≤1 egg per litre, additional health protection measures are required to safeguard the exposed children. These may include (i) anthelminthic treatment through mass chemotherapy campaigns or school-based chemotherapy programmes for helminthiasis control (see also section 4.2.2 on restricted irrigation), where health data indicate that helminth infections are prevalent; and/or (ii) the promotion of washing field vegetables in a weak detergent solution before consumption (see below). Alternatively, wastewater could be treated to the level of ≤0.1 egg per litre (see Box 5.2 in chapter 5).

An effective health protection measure for removing helminth eggs from the surface of crops eaten uncooked is washing the crop in a weak detergent solution and rinsing thoroughly with safe drinking-water. Helminth eggs are very "sticky," so they easily adhere to crop surfaces; the detergent solution releases them into the aqueous phase. This control measure reduces the number of eggs on the crop surface by 1–2 log units (B. Jiménez-Cisneros, personal communication, 2005). There is no specification for washing in a detergent and rinsing to obtain a 1–2 log reduction in the scientific literature, however, and in many cultures, the use of a detergent would rarely be complied with for certain crops such as lettuce or parsley (H. Shuval, personal communication, 2005).

The required helminth egg reduction to achieve the target of ≤1 egg per litre depends on the number of eggs in the raw wastewater. For example, if there are 10^3 eggs per litre in the raw wastewater, the required reduction is 3 log units; if there are 10^2, the required reduction is 2 log units; and if there are 10, the required reduction is 1 log unit (Table 4.4). Wastewater treatment processes to achieve, or partially achieve, these log unit reductions are described in chapter 5. If the number of helminth eggs in untreated wastewater is ≤1 per litre, then no additional health protection measures are required, as the target value is automatically achieved (this is the typical situation in most industrialized countries).

Table 4.4 shows examples of options for the reduction of helminth ova by two health protection measures and their associated verification requirements.

4.2.2 Restricted irrigation
Microbial reduction targets for viral, bacterial and protozoan pathogens
The Monte Carlo–QMRA results for labour-intensive restricted crop irrigation, based on the exposure scenario of involuntary soil ingestion, together with the relevant epidemiological evidence (chapter 3), show that in order to achieve the health-based target of ≤10^{-6} DALY per person per year for rotavirus, wastewater treatment is needed to achieve a reduction of the *E. coli* count by 4 log units (from 10^7–10^8 to 10^3–10^4 per 100 ml) (see Table 3.15 in chapter 3). Thus, for labour-intensive restricted irrigation, the health-based target is achieved by a 4 log unit pathogen reduction. This is illustrated by Option F in Figure 4.1. For highly mechanized agriculture, wastewater treatment to 10^5–10^6 *E. coli* per 100 ml is required (Table 3.14), i.e. a pathogen reduction of 3 log units, illustrated by Option G in Figure 4.1.

Option H in Figure 4.1 illustrates a typical single-household or institutional situation: minimal treatment in a septic tank (0.5 log unit pathogen reduction) followed by subsurface irrigation via the soil absorption system for the septic tank effluent. There is no contact between the crop and the pathogens in the septic tank effluent, so the subsurface irrigation system is credited with the remaining 6.5 log unit pathogen reduction required for root crops.

Table 4.4 Options for the reduction of helminth eggs by health protection measures for different helminth egg numbers in untreated wastewater and associated verification requirements

Health protection measure	Number of helminth eggs per litre of untreated wastewater	Required helminth egg reduction by treatment (log units)	Verification monitoring level (helminth eggs per litre of treated wastewater)[a]	Notes
Treatment	10^3	3	≤1	Treatment should be shown to achieve this egg quality reliably (see also Box 5.2).
	10^2	2	≤1	
	10	1	≤1	
	≤1	0	N/A	The target of ≤1 egg per litre is automatically achieved.
Treatment and produce washing	10^3	2	≤10	The reduction achieved by treatment is followed by a 1 log unit reduction by produce washing in a weak detergent solution and rinsing with clean water.[b]
	10^2	1	≤10	As above
	10	0	N/A	The required 1 log unit reduction is achieved by produce washing in a weak detergent solution and rinsing with clean water.[b]
	≤1	0	N/A	The target of ≤1 egg per litre is automatically achieved.

N/A, not applicable

[a] With waste stabilization ponds, the pond retention times can be used as a verification tool, as explained in Box 5.2. (Currently, there are no generally valid surrogate verification tools for other treatment processes, although it may be possible to develop them locally.)

[b] Valid only where this practice is common or where it can be successfully promoted and verified (see Table 4.3).

Microbial reduction targets for helminth eggs

The epidemiological evidence presented in chapter 3 provides the basis for developing a performance target for helminth eggs in restricted irrigation. The performance target for restricted irrigation is ≤1 helminth egg per litre of treated wastewater.

Epidemiological evidence from Mexico on *Ascaris* infection (section 3.2.2) shows that ≤1 egg per litre does not sufficiently protect children under the age of 15 who have exposure to wastewater-irrigated fields through either play or farming activities, although it does protect adult fieldworkers. Thus, when children under 15 are exposed by working or playing in wastewater-irrigated fields, additional health protection measures are required. In these circumstances, and where helminth infections are prevalent, anthelminthic treatment should be used as an additional risk management strategy. This may be delivered through school-based chemotherapy programmes for helminthiasis control (Montresor et al., 2002, 2005) or by periodic special treatment campaigns delivered by local health services in high-risk areas (especially where such children may not be attending schools). Where possible, such campaigns should also include a health promotion component to reduce exposure, for example, by emphasizing prevention of hand–soil contact through the use of gloves and appropriate tools and by hand washing with soap after contact with wastewater.

4.2.3 Localized irrigation

When localized irrigation (drip, trickle or bubbler irrigation) is used as a wastewater application technique, the log unit reductions for viral, bacterial and protozoan pathogens given in Table 4.3 should be used. In addition, when it is used to irrigate low-growing crops (i.e. those in partial contact with the soil), the microbial reduction target of ≤1 helminth egg per litre of treated wastewater should also be applied. However, when localized irrigation is used to irrigate high-growing crops (i.e. those with their harvested parts not in contact with the soil), specified performance targets for helminth egg concentrations are not necessary.

4.3 Verification monitoring

To ensure that health-based targets are being met, it is important to develop performance targets that can be monitored. There are three types of monitoring:

- Validation is the initial testing to prove that a system as a whole and its individual components are capable of meeting the performance targets and, thus, the health-based targets.
- Operational monitoring is the routine monitoring of parameters that can be measured rapidly (i.e. through tests that can be performed quickly, parameters measured online, or through visual inspection) to inform management decisions to prevent hazardous conditions from arising.
- Verification monitoring is done periodically to show that the system is working as intended. This type of monitoring usually requires more complicated or time-consuming tests that look at parameters such as bacterial indicators (*E. coli*) or helminth eggs.

Monitoring is further discussed in chapter 6. Verification monitoring requirements for unrestricted, restricted and localized irrigation are discussed below.

4.3.1 Wastewater treatment

As pathogen numbers in raw and treated wastewaters are not measured routinely (if at all), the performance of the wastewater treatment processes used to partially or wholly ensure $\leq 10^{-6}$ DALY per person per year cannot be determined on the basis of pathogen removal efficiency in the wastewater treatment plant. Therefore, monitoring to verify the microbiological performance of the treatment plant is done by determining the effluent numbers of a pathogen indicator bacterium such as *E. coli*. Table 4.5 lists for all the options in Figure 4.1 the numbers of *E. coli* in the treatment plant effluent that may be used as a verification tool to determine whether or not the required pathogen removal in the treatment plant is being achieved.

When advanced wastewater treatment is used as the sole health protection control measure (Option E in Figure 4.1), treatment plant performance may be verified using a selection of operational performance parameters, as shown in the footnote to Table 4.5 (State of California, 2001).

Table 4.5 Verification monitoring of wastewater treatment (*E. coli* numbers per 100 ml of treated wastewater) for the various levels of wastewater treatment in Options A–G in Figure 4.1

Type of irrigation	Option (Figure 4.1)	Required pathogen reduction by treatment (log units)	Verification monitoring level (*E. coli* per 100 ml)	Notes
Unrestricted	A	4	$\leq 10^3$	Root crops
	B	3	$\leq 10^4$	Leaf crops
	C	2	$\leq 10^5$	Drip irrigation of high-growing crops
	D	4	$\leq 10^3$	Drip irrigation of low-growing crops
	E	6 or 7	$\leq 10^1$ or $\leq 10^0$	Verification level depends on the requirements of the local regulatory agency[a]
Restricted	F	4	$\leq 10^4$	Labour-intensive agriculture (protective of adults and children under 15)
	G	3	$\leq 10^5$	Highly mechanized agriculture
	H	0.5	$\leq 10^6$	Pathogen removal in a septic tank

[a] For example, for secondary treatment, filtration and disinfection: five-day biochemical oxygen demand, <10 mg/l; turbidity, <2 nephelometric turbidity units; chlorine residual, 1 mg/l; pH, 6–9; and faecal coliforms, not detectable in 100 ml.

4.3.2 Other health protection measures

The health protection measures listed in Table 4.3, other than wastewater treatment (see section 4.3.1 above), also need to be monitored to ensure that they are in place and working as expected. Some of the health protection measures can be monitored by simple visual inspection (e.g. the types of crops being grown in wastewater irrigation areas, the type of wastewater application techniques being used, the use of protective clothing, the presence or absence of emergent vegetation in waste stabilization ponds or wastewater treatment and storage reservoirs); others will be more difficult to monitor (e.g. produce washing, disinfection, peeling and/or cooking at the household level). Verification of crop contamination levels at the point of harvest or at the point of sale will require laboratory analysis. As these health protection measures and their associated log unit pathogen reductions are central to health protection when wastewater treatment alone is not used to achieve the required total pathogen reduction of 6–7 log units, it is important to verify that they are in fact being used. Table 4.6 lists these minimum monitoring requirements.

4.4 Food exports

The rules that govern international trade in food were agreed during the Uruguay Round of Multilateral Trade Negotiations and apply to all members of the World Trade Organization (WTO). With regard to food safety, rules are set out in the Agreement on the Application of Sanitary and Phytosanitary Measures. According to this agreement, WTO members have the right to take legitimate measures to protect the life and health of their populations from hazards in food, provided that the measures are not unjustifiably restrictive of trade (WHO, 1999). The import of

Table 4.6 Minimum verification monitoring frequencies for health protection control measures

Health protection measures	Minimum verification monitoring frequency
Wastewater treatment	(a) Urban areas: one sample per fortnight for *E. coli* and one sample per month for helminth eggs
	(b) Rural areas: 1 sample every 3–6 months for helminth eggs
	Five-litre composite samples required for helminth eggs prepared from grab samples taken six times per day (further details given in Volume 5 of these Guidelines)
Localized (drip) irrigation with low and high rate-growing crops	Annual surveys to verify the irrigation method used and the types of crops grown
Spray irrigation (spray drift control and buffer zone)	Annual surveys to verify the spray drift control methods used and the extent of the buffer zone
Pathogen die-off	Annual local surveys to determine microbial quality of wastewater-irrigated crops at harvest and at selected points of retail sale
Produce washing, disinfection, peeling and cooking with water	Annual local surveys to verify occurrence at household level of these food preparation control measures and to assess the impact of food hygiene education programmes

contaminated vegetables has led to disease outbreaks in recipient countries. Moreover, pathogens can be (re)introduced into communities that have no natural immunity to them, resulting in large disease outbreaks (Frost et al., 1995; Kapperud et al., 1995). Guidelines for the international trade of wastewater-irrigated food products should be based on sound scientific risk management principles.

WHO Guidelines for the safe use of wastewater in agriculture are based on a risk analysis approach that is recognized as the fundamental methodology underlying the development of food safety standards that both provide adequate health protection and facilitate trade in food. Adherence to the recommended WHO Guidelines for exports of wastewater-irrigated food products will help to ensure the international trade of safe food products. EUREPGAP, a private sector European organization for sustainable agriculture and the certification of food imports into Europe, prohibits the use of untreated wastewater for crop irrigation but accepts the use of wastewater treated to the guideline values specified in the second edition of these Guidelines (EUREPGAP, 2004).

4.5 National standards: variations from $\leq 10^{-6}$ DALY per person per year

The performance targets developed for unrestricted and restricted irrigation in section 4.2 provide "full" health protection (i.e. they achieve the health-based target of $\leq 10^{-6}$ DALY per person per year). However, it is realized that some countries may wish to set different standards based on local circumstances. For example, some developing countries may not be able to afford the cost of wastewater treatment, even for restricted irrigation. Wastewater treatment may be considered to be of a low priority if the local incidence of diarrhoeal disease is high and other water supply, sanitation and hygiene promotion interventions are more cost-effective in controlling transmission. In such circumstances, it is recommended that, initially, a national standard is established for a locally appropriate level of tolerable additional burden of disease based on the local incidence of diarrhoeal diseases — for example, $\leq 10^{-5}$ or $\leq 10^{-4}$ DALY per person per year.

This initial standard should then be made progressively more stringent so that it eventually reaches the health-based target of $\leq 10^{-6}$ DALY per person per year (see Anderson et al., 2001; von Sperling & Fattal, 2001). It may also need to be accompanied by an enforced legal prohibition on children working in fields irrigated by raw or inadequately treated wastewater (initially, this might refer to children under, for example, 10 years of age; over time, this could be extended to children under 15). The health basis of such a prohibition should be clearly explained to those affected by it, in particular subsistence farmers with children under the age of 10 or 15. Additional health protection measures for reducing the adverse health impacts of the currently widespread practice of crop irrigation with raw wastewater are described in chapter 5.

Some countries may wish to focus on preventing the transmission of bacterial infections through wastewater irrigation, where immunity to viral infections develops at a young age and other transmission routes are more important. For example, the main risk factors for rotavirus infection are person-to-person contact, absence of breastfeeding and hygiene related to use of babies' bottles, and immunity is developed by the age of five in most people (although infections do occur in adults). The risk of infection for *Campylobacter* is 10^{-4} per person per year (Table 4.2). However, QMRA has indicated that the water quality associated with a *Campylobacter* infection risk of 1×10^{-4} per person per year is 1 log unit less than that for a rotavirus infection risk of 1×10^{-3}. Thus, in the case of unrestricted irrigation, the required wastewater quality would be 10^4–10^5 *E. coli* per 100 ml, rather than 10^3–10^4 *E. coli* per 100 ml (see Table 3.19 in chapter 3). In such circumstances, the verification monitoring level would also change by 1 log unit, making the level for unrestricted irrigation of leafy crops $\leq 10^5$ *E. coli* per 100 ml. The values for restricted irrigation would change in a similar way (see Tables 3.14–3.16).

Some developing countries may also wish to set an initially less stringent performance target for helminth eggs if their local prevalence of helminthiases is high and other control interventions are likely to be more cost-effective in the short term. For example, the initial target might be ≤ 10 or ≤ 5 eggs per litre of treated wastewater.

Similarly, an industrialized country that already has a more stringent national health-based target (e.g. equivalent to $\leq 10^{-7}$ DALY per person per year) or other objectives (e.g. environmental regulations) may wish to keep them — for example, where a lower tolerable risk of infection or disease is already used and where adequate wastewater treatment plants already exist and their reliable operation is assured.

4.6 Chemicals

4.6.1 Health-based targets

To derive the numerical limits for the maximum tolerable pollutant concentration in wastewater-irrigated soils, the process starts with establishing the acceptable daily human intake (ADI) for a pollutant. It then quantitatively backtracks the pollutant transport through various environmental exposure routes to arrive at a tolerable pollutant concentration in the soil. Human exposure to pollutants applied to soils through wastewater irrigation may take place through eight pathways (USEPA, 1992), as follows:

1. wastewater → soil → plant → human;
2. wastewater → soil → human;
3. wastewater → soil → plant → animal → human;
4. wastewater → soil → animal → human;
5. wastewater → soil → airborne particulate → human;
6. wastewater → soil → surface runoff → surface water → human;
7. wastewater → soil → vadose zone → groundwater → human;
8. wastewater → soil → atmosphere → human.

To obtain preliminary numerical limits in wastewater-irrigated soils, a simplified approach was adopted. Instead of assessing all of the exposure routes, WHO considered only (a) the food-chain transfer of pollutants via the wastewater → soil → plant → human route and (b) the pollutant intake from the consumption of grain, vegetable, root/tuber crops and fruit. Food-chain transfer is the primary route of human exposure to environmental pollutants. Based on the global diet, the daily intake of grains/cereals, vegetables, root/tuber crops and fruit accounts for approximately 75% of daily adult food consumption (Gleick, 2000). The exposure scenario assumed that most exposed individuals were the adult residents (60 kg of body weight) of a land application area whose entire consumption of grain, vegetables, root/tuber crops and fruit was produced from wastewater-irrigated soils and that their daily intake of pollutants from this consumption accounted for 50% of the ADI. The remaining 50% of the ADI was credited to other exposure routes (e.g. drinking-water, cigarettes, etc.).

Based on the assumption that food-chain transfer is the primary route of exposure to potentially hazardous pollutants in the wastewater, WHO derived numerical limits defining the maximum permissible pollutant concentrations in soils for a set of organic and inorganic pollutants. These maximum permissible health-related pollutant concentrations in the receiving soils are summarized in Table 4.7. They define safe concentrations in the soil above which the transfer of pollutants to people via the food-chain may occur. For inorganic elements, their concentrations in wastewater-irrigated soils will slowly rise with each successive wastewater application. However, for many of the organic pollutants, the likelihood is small that they will accumulate in the soil to their computed threshold concentrations because their typical concentrations in wastewaters are very low.

Table 4.7 Maximum tolerable soil concentrations of various toxic chemicals based on human health protection

Chemical	Soil concentration (mg/kg)
Element	
Antimony	36
Arsenic	8
Barium[a]	302
Beryllium[a]	0.2
Boron[a]	1.7
Cadmium	4
Fluorine	635
Lead	84
Mercury	7

Table 4.7 (continued)

Chemical	Soil concentration (mg/kg)
Molybdenum[a]	0.6
Nickel	107
Selenium	6
Silver	3
Thallium[a]	0.3
Vanadium[a]	47
Organic compound	
Aldrin	0.48
Benzene	0.14
Chlordane	3
Chlorobenzene	211
Chloroform	0.47
2,4-D	0.25
DDT	1.54
Dichlorobenzene	15
Dieldrin	0.17
Dioxins	0.000 12
Heptachlor	0.18
Hexachlorobenzene	1.40
Lindane	12
Methoxychlor	4.27
PAHs (as benzo[*a*]pyrene)	16
PCBs	0.89
Pentachlorophenol	14
Phthalate	13 733
Pyrene	41
Styrene	0.68
2,4,5-T	3.82
Tetrachloroethane	1.25
Tetrachloroethylene	0.54
Toluene	12
Toxaphene	0.0013
Trichloroethane	0.68

[a] The computed numerical limits for these elements are within the ranges that are typical for soils.

4.6.2 Physicochemical quality of treated wastewaters for plant growth requirements

To accommodate plant growth requirements, the physicochemical quality of treated wastewaters used for crop irrigation should comply with the guideline values set by the FAO (Ayers & Westcot, 1985; Tanji & Kielen, 2002). This information is summarized in Annex 1.

5
HEALTH PROTECTION MEASURES

As described in chapter 4, the health-based target of a tolerable additional burden of disease of $\leq 10^{-6}$ DALY per person per year can be achieved when treated wastewater is used for crop irrigation, by a combination of health protection measures that produces an overall pathogen reduction of 6–7 log units (Figure 4.1; Table 4.3). These control measures include:

- crop restriction;
- wastewater application technique;
- pathogen die-off between last irrigation and consumption;
- food preparation measures (washing, disinfecting, peeling, cooking);
- human exposure control;
- wastewater treatment.

The selection of health protection measures by planners and designers of wastewater use schemes can be based on several factors, including the current wastewater treatment infrastructure and the products that will be grown. For new schemes, planning for crop restriction might be a desirable option, as the target of $\leq 10^{-6}$ DALY per person per year is achieved by a pathogen reduction of only 2–3 log units compared with the 6–7 log unit reduction required for unrestricted irrigation (Figure 4.1); it is therefore a lower-cost option.

The feasibility and efficacy of any combination of these health protection measures will depend on several factors, which must be carefully considered before any combination of them is put into practice. These factors include:

- availability of resources (labour, funds, land, water);
- existing social and agricultural practices;
- market demand for wastewater-irrigated food and non-food crops;
- existing patterns of excreta-related disease;
- institutional capacity and jurisdiction to ensure the efficacy of selected health protection measures (e.g. ability to (a) ensure that wastewater treatment is effective in reducing pathogens to the extent required; and (b) promote effectively washing or disinfection of wastewater-irrigated produce).

These health protection measures are effective against the pathogens and some chemicals present in the wastewater that are the primary health hazards associated with the agricultural use of wastewater. There are, however, secondary risks that may arise from the creation of habitats that facilitate the survival and breeding of vectors and a subsequent increase in the transmission of vector-borne diseases in wastewater-irrigated areas. Conducting an analysis of any existing or proposed wastewater irrigation system will identify the key risk points, and this is an important step in identifying which health protection measures are likely to be appropriate (see chapter 6). Health impact assessment (Annex 3) will also help to identify health hazards and risk factors that may arise due to wastewater use in agriculture; this will provide a context for the formulation of a public health action plan.

The health protection measures listed above are discussed in detail in sections 5.1–5.6. Their application when untreated wastewater is used for crop irrigation is presented in section 5.7.

5.1 Crop restriction

Restricted irrigation produces many useful and profitable crops, including (a) non-food crops (e.g. cotton and "biodiesel" crops such as jojoba, jatropha and rapeseed); (b) food crops that are processed before consumption (wheat); and (c) food crops that have to be cooked (potatoes, rice). The vulnerable group includes those who work in wastewater-irrigated fields (and also, if spray or sprinkler irrigation is used, nearby residents; see section 5.2). Crop consumers are protected because they either do not eat the foods or eat them only after extensive processing and/or cooking, which inactivate the pathogens. As shown in Figure 4.1 and section 4.2.2, the health-based target of $\leq 10^{-6}$ DALY per fieldworker per year can be met with a 2 or 3 log unit pathogen reduction (depending on whether children under the age of 15 are exposed or not), compared with the 6–7 log unit reduction required for unrestricted irrigation.

Crop restriction requires, of course, that farmers use only wastewater that has been treated to the quality required for unrestricted irrigation to irrigate food crops that are eaten uncooked. Thus, restricted irrigation is feasible where:

- a law-abiding society and/or strong law enforcement exists;
- a public body controls allocation of the wastes and has the legal authority to require that crop restrictions be adhered to;
- an irrigation project has strong central management;
- there is adequate demand for the crops allowed under crop restriction, and where they produce a reasonable profit;
- there is little market pressure in favour of excluded crops.

It is important that planners and designers of restricted irrigation schemes engage with local farmers early in the planning process to consult them and determine what "restricted crops" can be grown at a reasonable profit. They must clearly understand the difference between restricted and unrestricted irrigation (including the different wastewater qualities used for each), and they must be aware of the health consequences that will occur if they irrigate food crops that are eaten uncooked with wastewater treated only to the level for restricted irrigation.

Examples of successful crop restriction schemes are found in India, Mexico, Peru and Chile (Blumenthal et al., 2000b; Buechler & Devi, 2003). In Chile, the use of crop restriction, when implemented with a general hygiene education programme, reduced the transmission of cholera from the consumption of raw wastewater–irrigated vegetables by 90% (Monreal, 1993). Experience from Hyderabad, India, indicates that restricted irrigation is not synonymous with restricted farmer income: two of the most profitable wastewater-irrigated crops are para grass (used to feed water buffalo) and jasmine flowers (used for flavouring tea) (Buechler & Devi, 2003).

5.2 Wastewater application techniques

The choice of wastewater application method can impact the health status of farm workers, consumers and nearby communities (Table 5.1).

5.2.1 Flood and furrow irrigation

Fieldworkers and their families are at the highest risk when furrow or flood irrigation techniques are used. This is especially true when protective clothing (i.e. boots, shoes, gloves) is not worn and earth is moved by hand (Blumenthal et al., 2000b). However, wastewater treatment to achieve a pathogen reduction of 2–3 log units protects fieldworkers (sections 4.2.3 and 5.6).

Table 5.1 Selection of wastewater application techniques based on health protection

Irrigation technique	Factors affecting choice	Special measures for wastewater
Flood	Lowest cost Exact levelling not required	Thorough protection for fieldworkers, crop handlers and consumers
Furrow	Low cost Levelling may be needed	Protection for fieldworkers, possibly for crop handlers and consumers
Spray and sprinkler	Medium water use efficiency Levelling not required Advanced sprinklers that reduce crop contamination and potential contamination of local communities have been developed that can reduce exposure to pathogens by 1 log unit	Some crops, especially tree fruits, are prone to more contamination Minimum distance of 50–100 m from houses and roads Anaerobic wastewaters should not be used because of odour nuisance New technologies reduce spray drift and may be able to reduce crop contamination by better targeting
Subsurface and localized (drip, trickle and bubbler)	High cost High water use efficiency Higher yields Potential for significant reduction of crop contamination Localized irrigation systems and subsurface irrigation can substantially reduce exposure to pathogens by 2–6 log units	Localized irrigation: selection of non-clogging emitters; filtration to prevent clogging of emitters

5.2.2 Spray and sprinkler irrigation

Spray and sprinkler irrigation have the highest potential to spread contamination onto crop surfaces and affect nearby communities. Bacteria and viruses (but not usually helminth eggs or protozoan (oo)cysts) can be transmitted through aerosols to nearby communities. Where spray or sprinkler irrigation is used with wastewater, it may be necessary to set up a buffer zone (e.g. 50–100 m from houses and roads) to prevent adverse health impacts on local communities. Setting up an adequate buffer zone is equivalent to a 1 log unit pathogen reduction (see Table 4.3 in chapter 4) (NRMMC & EPHCA, 2005). Spray drift away from the site of application can be reduced by using techniques such as low-throw sprinklers, micro-sprinklers, part-circle sprinklers (180 degrees inward throw), tree/shrub screens planted at field borders and anemometer switching systems (NRMMC & EPHCA, 2005).

5.2.3 Localized irrigation

Localized irrigation techniques (e.g. bubbler, drip, trickle) offer farm workers the most health protection because the wastewater is applied directly to the plants. Although these techniques are generally the most expensive to implement, low-cost drip irrigation systems have recently been adopted by some farmers in Cape Verde and India (Kay, 2001; Postel, 2001; FAO, 2002). The benefits of these systems in terms of reduced (waste)water usage and higher crop yields convinced many private farmers in Cape Verde to drip-irrigate their crops. Further research on viable approaches using suitable local materials (e.g. bamboo) may facilitate greater uptake of this technology in various low-resource settings.

Localized irrigation is estimated to provide an additional pathogen reduction of 2–4 log units, depending on whether or not the harvested part of the crop is in contact with the ground (see Table 4.3) (NRMMC & EPHCA, 2005).

The emitters used in drip irrigation can block if the suspended solids content of the wastewater is high. Emitter blockage also occurs as a result of soil-based algae migrating to the emitters, as this is where the wastewater nutrients are released. Algae from waste stabilization ponds do not usually block emitters, although care is required to choose an emitter that does not block easily (Taylor et al., 1995; Capra & Scicolone, 2004).

5.2.4 Cessation of irrigation

Vaz da Costa Vargas, Bastos & Mara (1996) showed that cessation of irrigation with wastewater for one to two weeks prior to harvest can be effective in reducing crop contamination by providing time for pathogen die-off (section 5.3). Enforcing withholding periods is likely to be difficult, however, in unregulated circumstances, because many vegetables (especially lettuce and other leafy vegetables) need watering nearly until harvest to increase their market value. However, it may be possible with some fodder crops that do not have to be harvested at the peak of their freshness (Blumenthal et al., 2000b). Alternatively, crops could be irrigated from non-contaminated water sources (where available) after the cessation of wastewater use until harvest.

5.3 Pathogen die-off before consumption

The interval between final irrigation and consumption reduces pathogens (bacteria, protozoa and viruses) by approximately 1 log unit per day (Petterson & Ashbolt, 2003). The precise value depends on climatic conditions, with more rapid pathogen die-off (approximately 2 log units per day) in hot, dry weather and less in cool or wet weather without much direct sunlight (approximately 0.5 log unit per day). This reduction is extremely reliable and should be taken into account when selecting the combination of wastewater treatment and other health protection measures (see Figure 4.1 in chapter 4). Helminth eggs can remain viable on crop surfaces for up to two months, although few survive beyond approximately 30 days (Strauss, 1996) (see also section 3.1.1).

5.4 Food preparation measures

Vigorous washing of rough-surfaced salad crops (e.g. lettuce, parsley) and vegetables eaten uncooked in tap water reduces bacteria by at least 1 log unit; for smooth-surfaced salad crops (e.g. cucumbers, tomatoes), the reduction is approximately 2 log units (Brackett, 1987; Beuchat, 1998; Lang et al., 2004). Washing in a disinfectant solution (commonly a hypochlorite solution) and rinsing in tap water can reduce pathogens by 1–2 log units. Washing in a detergent (e.g. washing-up liquid) solution and rinsing in tap water can reduce helminth egg numbers by 1–2 log units (B. Jiménez-Cisneros, personal communication, 2005).

Peeling fruits and root vegetables reduces pathogens by at least 2 log units. Cooking vegetables achieves an essentially complete reduction (5–6 log units) of pathogens.

These reductions are extremely reliable and should always be taken into account when selecting the combination of wastewater treatment and other health-based control measures (see Figure 4.1). Effective hygiene education and promotion programmes will be required to inform local food handlers (in markets, in the home and in restaurants and food kiosks) how and why they should wash wastewater-irrigated produce effectively with water or disinfectant and/or detergent solutions.

5.5 Human exposure control

5.5.1 Fieldworkers

Agricultural fieldworkers are at high potential, and often actual, risk of parasitic infections. However, a recent case–control study in Viet Nam of wastewater-irrigated "wet" rice culture shows that farmers engaged in wastewater-fed rice culture have no higher risk of helminth infections than farmers using river water for irrigation (Trang et al., in press). Such risks can be reduced, even eliminated, by the use of less-contaminating irrigation methods (section 5.2) and by the use of appropriate protective clothing (i.e. shoes or boots for fieldworkers and gloves for crop handlers). These health protection measures have not been quantified in terms of pathogen exposure reduction but are expected to have an important positive effect. This is especially true for wearing shoes or boots where there is a risk of hookworm or schistosomiasis transmission. Fieldworkers should be provided with access to sanitation facilities and adequate water for drinking and hygienic purposes in order to avoid the consumption of, and any contact with, wastewater. Similarly, safe water should be provided at markets for washing and "freshening" produce. A study conducted in Peru indicated that wastewater-irrigated crops with acceptable levels of bacteria at the farm were frequently recontaminated in the market (Castro de Esparza & Vargas, 1990, cited in Peasey et al., 2000).

Effective hygiene promotion programmes are almost always needed (Blumenthal et al., 2000b). These should target fieldworkers, produce handlers, vendors and consumers. Hand washing with soap should be emphasized. It may be possible to link hygiene promotion to agricultural extension activities or other health programmes (e.g. immunization programmes).

The risk of cattle ingesting helminth eggs from the soil is high, because grazing cattle may ingest 1–18% of their dry matter intake as soil and sheep as much as 30%, depending on the management and supply of grass (Cabaret et al., 2002). Although *Taenia* eggs have been known to survive for several months on grazing land, the risk of bovine cysticercosis is greatly reduced by ceasing wastewater application at least two weeks before cattle are allowed to graze (Feachem et al., 1983). Tapeworm transmission can be controlled by good meat inspection, provided that animals are slaughtered only in recognized abattoirs where all carcasses are inspected and all infected carcasses rejected.

Precautions against schistosomiasis transmission in endemic areas should also be taken. For example, fieldworkers should be given boots to wear when working in irrigation canals. On large commercial wastewater irrigation schemes, molluscicides may be added to the treated wastewater as it leaves the treatment works.

5.5.2 Consumers

The food preparation measures detailed in section 5.4 protect consumers, but not those preparing the food, who are best protected by exposure control techniques such as rigorous personal and domestic hygiene, frequent hand washing with soap, the use of separate areas for food preparation and the subsequent handling of washed, disinfected and cooked food. Effective hygiene education and promotion are required.

5.5.3 Chemotherapy and immunization

Immunization against helminth infections and most diarrhoeal diseases is currently not feasible. However, for highly exposed groups, immunization against typhoid may be worth considering. Tourists visiting areas where wastewater is used frequently to irrigate crops should be vaccinated against typhoid and hepatitis A virus to give them more protection against these diseases.

Additional protection may be provided by the availability of adequate medical facilities to treat diarrhoeal disease and by regular chemotherapy. This might include chemotherapeutic control of intense helminth infections in children and control of anaemia in both children and adults, especially women and post-menarche girls. Chemotherapy must be reapplied at regular intervals to be effective. The frequency required to keep worm burdens at a low level (e.g. as low as in the rest of the population) depends on the intensity of the transmission, but chemotherapy may be required 2–3 times a year for children living in endemic areas (Montresor et al., 2002). Albonico et al. (1995) found that reinfection with helminths could return to pretreatment levels within six months of a mass chemotherapy campaign if the prevailing conditions did not change.

Chemotherapy and immunization cannot normally be considered as adequate strategies to protect fieldworkers and their families exposed to raw wastewater (section 5.7). However, where such workers are organized within structured situations, such as government or company farms, chemotherapy and immunization could be beneficial as palliative measures, pending improvement in the quality of the wastewater used or the adoption of other health-based control measures (e.g. protective clothing).

For schistosomiasis, a chemotherapy programme targeted at the highest-risk populations is recommended. In high-prevalence situations, WHO suggests that school-age children be treated once per year. Community-directed treatment for other high-risk groups (e.g. agricultural fieldworkers) should be made available. Where the prevalence of schistosomiasis is moderate, school-age children should be treated once every two years. In communities where schistosomiasis prevalence is low, school-age children should be treated twice during primary schooling (once at the beginning and again on leaving) (WHO, 2002).

5.6 Wastewater treatment

Wastewater treatment processes are described in this section primarily with respect to their ability to remove excreted pathogens, rather than to describe their design and operation, which are detailed in some recent texts (e.g. Metcalf & Eddy, Inc., 2003; Mara, 2004; Ludwig et al., 2005; von Sperling & Chernicharo, 2005). Validation, operational and verification monitoring of wastewater treatment processes are described in chapter 6. A comprehensive review of pathogen reduction in the environment, including removal during wastewater treatment, is given in Asano (1998) and Feachem et al. (1983). Typical ranges of pathogen removals in various wastewater treatment processes are given in Table 5.2.

A rigorous costing methodology for comparing and selecting wastewater treatment processes, which includes the cost of the land area required, is given by Arthur (1983). The advantages and disadvantages of various wastewater treatment processes are listed in Table 5.3.

Table 5.2 Log unit reduction or inactivation of excreted pathogens achieved by selected wastewater treatment processes

Treatment process	Log unit pathogen removals[a]			
	Viruses	Bacteria	Protozoan (oo)cysts	Helminth eggs
Low-rate biological processes				
Waste stabilization ponds	1–4	1–6	1–4	1–3[b]
Wastewater storage and treatment reservoirs	1–4	1–6	1–4	1–3[b]
Constructed wetlands	1–2	0.5–3	0.5–2	1–3[b]
High-rate processes				
Primary treatment				
Primary sedimentation	0–1	0–1	0–1	0–<1[b]
Chemically enhanced primary treatment	1–2	1–2	1–2	1–3[b]
Anaerobic upflow sludge blanket reactors	0–1	0.5–1.5	0–1	0.5–1[b]
Secondary treatment				
Activated sludge + secondary sedimentation	0–2	1–2	0–1	1–<2[b]
Trickling filters + secondary sedimentation	0–2	1–2	0–1	1–2[c]
Aerated lagoon + settling pond	1–2	1–2	0–1	1–3[c]
Tertiary treatment				
Coagulation/flocculation	1–3	0–1	1–3	2[b]
High-rate granular or slow-rate sand filtration	1–3	0–3	0–3	1–3[b]
Dual-media filtration	1–3	0–1	1–3	2–3[b,d]
Membranes	2.5–>6	3.5–>6	>6	>3[b,d]
Disinfection				
Chlorination (free chlorine)	1–3	2–6	0–1.5	0–<1[b]
Ozonation	3–6	2–6	1–2	0–2[e]
Ultraviolet radiation	1–>3	2–>4	>3	0[e]

Sources: Feachem et al. (1983); Schwartzbrod et al. (1989); Sobsey (1989); El-Gohary et al. (1993); Rivera et al. (1995); Rose et al. (1996, 1997); Strauss (1996); Landa, Capella & Jiménez (1997); Clancy et al. (1998); National Research Council (1998); Yates & Gerba (1998); Karimi, Vickers & Harasick (1999); Lazarova et al. (2000); Jiménez et al. (2001); Jiménez & Chávez (2002); Jiménez (2003, 2005); von Sperling et al. (2003); Mara (2004); Rojas-Valencia et al. (2004); WHO (2004a); NRMMC & EPHCA (2005).

[a] The log unit reductions are log_{10} unit reductions defined as log_{10} (initial pathogen concentration/final pathogen concentration). Thus, a 1 log unit reduction = 90% reduction; a 2 log unit reduction = 99% reduction; a 3 log unit reduction = 99.9% reduction; and so on.

[b] Data from full-scale plants.

[c] Theoretical efficiency based on removal mechanisms.

[d] Data from tests with up to 2 log units initial content; removal may be greater than that reported.

[e] Data from laboratory tests.

Table 5.3 Advantages and disadvantages of different wastewater treatment processes

Treatment	Advantages	Disadvantages[a]
Low-rate biological systems		
Waste stabilization ponds, wastewater storage and treatment reservoirs	Effective at reducing pathogen concentrations (all types of pathogens) Low costs of construction, operation and maintenance Simplicity of operation and maintenance Produce little sludge with low helminth ova content Work well in warm climates with medium to low evaporation No use of electrical energy for operation Help to reconcile wastewater production with water irrigation demand because they can store water for use at peak demand times	Hydraulic short-circuiting may reduce pathogen removal efficiency Algae in effluents may interfere with irrigation application Require large amounts of land (especially in temperate environments) Can facilitate vector breeding if not properly maintained High evaporation in arid climates leads to loss of water resources and increased effluent salinity
Constructed wetlands	Effective in reducing pathogen concentrations — medium bacterial and viral removal efficiency Low cost, low complexity Relatively simple operation and maintenance requirements Require no electricity May improve environment for other species (e.g. birds)	Pathogen removal variable, depending upon a variety of factors Different designs/plants needed in different settings High evapotranspiration in arid climates leads to loss of water resources and increased effluent salinity May facilitate vector breeding Wildlife excreta may cause deterioration of effluent quality
High-rate processes		
Primary sedimentation	Low cost Simple technology	Low pathogen removal
Chemically enhanced primary treatment	Improves primary sedimentation at low cost Low area requirement High helminth egg removal efficiency Produces effluents suitable for agricultural needs	Produces more sludge than normal primary sedimentation Need to treat the sludge produced to inactivate pathogens Need to use chemicals
Activated sludge or trickling filters + secondary sedimentation + disinfection	Technology widely available and well understood Performance can be optimized for good pathogen removal	High cost and complexity Need trained staff Require electricity Produce large volumes of sludge, which need to be handled, treated and disposed of Need to treat the sludge produced to inactivate pathogens Sludge bulking may increase helminth egg numbers in the effluent

Table 5.3 (continued)

Treatment	Advantages	Disadvantages[a]
Upflow anaerobic sludge blanket reactor	Low cost Medium helminth egg removal efficiency	Effluent can cause odour problems Needs trained staff Sludge needs digestion and/or treatment to inactivate pathogens
Aerated lagoon + settling pond	Technology widely available and well understood Performance can be optimized for good pathogen removal No need for primary sedimentation	Require electricity Require larger land area than other high-rate processes Less expensive and complex than other high-rate processes Sludge needs to be treated to inactivate pathogens
Coagulation, flocculation and sedimentation	Improve virus and other pathogen removal/inactivation efficiency Low additional cost	Increase sludge production Sludge needs to be treated to inactivate pathogens
High-rate granular or slow-rate sand filtration	Improves pathogen removal Well understood technology Low additional cost	Needs careful management to optimize performance Slow-rate filters require more space Sludge needs to be treated to inactivate pathogens
Dual-media filtration	When used after primary treatment, efficiently removes protozoan (oo)cysts and helminth eggs When used after secondary treatment, improves pathogen removal Well understood technology Low additional cost	Low efficiency of bacterial and viral removals Needs careful management to optimize performance
Chlorination (free chlorine)	Lowest-cost disinfection method Well understood technology Effective inactivation of bacteria and viruses	Needs pretreatment to be efficient Low efficiency of protozoan and helminth inactivation Creates disinfection by-products Hazardous chemical
Ozone disinfection	Effective inactivation of bacteria, viruses and some protozoa	Effective where organic matter is low Higher cost and complexity than chlorination Low efficiency of protozoan and helminth inactivation Needs to be generated on site Production of hazardous by-products
Ultraviolet disinfection	Effective in inactivating bacteria, viruses and some protozoa Low cost No toxic chemicals used or produced	Effective only in effluents with low suspended solids content and high transmittance Does not inactivate helminth eggs Performance can be reduced by particulate matter and biofilm formation Needs good maintenance of lamps

Table 5.3 (continued)

Treatment	Advantages	Disadvantages[a]
Primary sedimentation + membrane bioreactors	Remove all pathogens	Complex
		Expensive
		Sludge needs to be treated to inactivate pathogens
		Membrane fouling

Sources: Feachem et al. (1983); Schwartzbrod et al. (1989); Sobsey (1989); Rivera et al. (1995); Rose et al. (1996, 1997); Strauss (1996); Landa, Capella & Jiménez (1997); Asano & Levine (1998); Clancy et al. (1998); National Research Council (1998); Yates & Gerba (1998); Karimi, Vickers & Harasick (1999); Lazarova et al. (2000); Jiménez et al. (2001); Jiménez & Chávez (2002); Jiménez (2003, 2005); Metcalf & Eddy, Inc. (2003); von Sperling et al. (2003); Mara (2004); Rojas-Valencia et al. (2004); WHO (2004a); NRMMC & EPHCA (2005); von Sperling & Chernicharo (2005).

[a] Many of these disadvantages can be minimized by careful engineering design and good operation and maintenance.

Two types of treatment systems are described in this section:

- low-rate biological systems: mostly pond-based systems with long retention times;
- high-rate processes: mostly engineered structures with short retention times (i.e. high flow rates).

5.6.1 Low-rate biological systems
Waste stabilization ponds

Waste stabilization ponds are shallow basins that use natural factors such as sunlight, temperature, sedimentation, biodegradation, etc., to treat wastewater (Jiménez, 2003; Mara, 2004). Water treatment systems made up of stabilization ponds usually consist of anaerobic, facultative and maturation ponds linked in series. For optimal performance, the ponds should be designed in such a way as to minimize or eliminate hydraulic short-circuiting. In tropical environments (20–30 °C), well designed and properly operated and maintained waste stabilization pond systems can achieve a 2–4 log unit removal of viruses, a 3–6 log unit removal of bacterial pathogens, a 1–2 log unit removal of protozoan (oo)cysts and a 3 log unit removal of helminth eggs; the precise values depend on the number of ponds in series and their retention times (Mara & Silva, 1986; Oragui et al., 1987; Grimason et al., 1993; see Mara, 2004, for further details on waste stabilization pond design for pathogen removal).

Protozoan (oo)cysts and helminth eggs are removed by sedimentation (and thus remain in the pond sludge). Viruses are removed by adsorption onto solids, including algae (if these solids settle, the adsorbed viruses also remain in the pond sludge). Bacteria are removed or inactivated by several mechanisms, including temperature, pH values above 9.4 (induced by rapid algal photosynthesis) and a combination of high light intensity (>450 nm wavelength) and high dissolved oxygen concentrations (Curtis, Mara & Silva, 1992).

The design of waste stabilization ponds for helminth egg and *E. coli* removal is outlined in Box 5.1; both procedures are very reliable, and, as explained in the box, measured values of the mean hydraulic retention times in waste stabilization ponds can be used as a simple surrogate estimation of the number of helminth eggs in the final effluent (i.e. to check compliance with the microbial reduction target for helminths of ≤1 egg per litre). Evaporation should always be taken into account in waste stabilization pond design (Mara, 2004).

Box 5.1 Design of waste stabilization ponds for helminth egg and *E. coli* reduction

Helminth eggs

The design equation of Ayres et al. (1992b) is used:

$$R = 100[1 - 0.41\exp(-0.49\theta + 0.00850\theta^2)]$$

where R is the percent egg reduction in an anaerobic, facultative or maturation pond; and θ is the retention time in the pond (in days). Thus, for a series of ponds:

$$E_e = E_i(1 - r_a)(1 - r_f)(1 - r_m)^n$$

where E_e and E_i are the numbers of helminth eggs per litre of the final effluent and the raw wastewater, respectively; $r = R/100$; the subscripts a, f and m refer to the anaerobic, facultative and maturation ponds; and n is the number of equally sized maturation ponds.

The retention time in a pond defines the helminth egg reduction in it. Thus, if the flow (Q, m³/day) into a pond is measured regularly during the irrigation season, and since its retention time (θ, days) is then known (= V/Q, where V is the pond volume, m³), R can be calculated. If this is done for every pond in the series, and provided E_i is determined on every occasion the flow is measured, E_e can be determined.

An alternative approach is to calculate the total egg reduction in the waste stabilization pond series (R_T), as follows:

$$R_T = 100[1 - (1 - r_a)(1 - r_f)(1 - r_m)^n]$$

As E_e should be ≤1 egg per litre (Table 4.4), then the maximum number of eggs in the raw wastewater ($E_{i(max)}$) consistent with $E_e = 1$ is given by:

$$E_{i(max)} = E_e(1 - r_T)^{-1} = (1 - r_T)^{-1}$$

where $r_T = R_T/100$. If this calculated value of $E_{i(max)}$ is more than the known value of E_i, then the waste stabilization pond system can be safely assumed to be producing a final effluent with ≤1 helminth egg per litre. Thus, routine monitoring for helminth eggs is not required; it would be sufficient to determine E_i on a few occasions at the start of every irrigation season.

E. coli
The equations of Marais (1966) are used. For a single pond:

$$N_e = \frac{N_i}{1 + k_{B(T)}\theta}$$

$$k_{B(T)} = 2.6(1.19)^{T-20}$$

where N_e and N_i are the numbers of *E. coli* per 100 ml of the pond effluent and influent, respectively; $k_{B(T)}$ is the first-order rate constant for *E. coli* reduction at T °C in a completely mixed reactor (/day); θ is the mean hydraulic retention time in the pond (days); and T is the design temperature (°C).

For a series of anaerobic, facultative and maturation ponds, the first equation above becomes (since the effluent of one pond is the influent to the next):

Box 5.1 (continued)

$$N_e = \frac{N_i}{(1 + k_{B(T)}\theta_a)(1 + k_{B(T)}\theta_f)(1 + k_{B(T)}\theta_m)^n}$$

where N_e and N_i are now the *E. coli* numbers per 100 ml of the final effluent and the raw wastewater, respectively; the subscripts a, f and m refer to the anaerobic, facultative and maturation ponds; and n is the number of equally sized maturation ponds. For use in design, this equation is rewritten as:

$$\theta_m = \{[N_i/N_e(1 + k_{B(T)}\theta_a)(1 + k_{B(T)}\theta_f)(1 + k_{B(T)}\theta_{m1})]^{1/n} - 1\}/k_{B(T)}$$

This form of the equation enables the waste stabilization pond series to be easily designed for the required number of *E. coli* per 100 ml of final effluent (N_e) (Figure 4.1; Table 4.5). It is solved first for $n = 1$, then for $n = 2$ and so on, until the calculated value of θ_m is <3 days (the minimum permissible retention time in a maturation pond). The designer then selects the most appropriate combination of n and θ_m (i.e. the one that has the least overall retention time and therefore the least land area requirement).

Waste stabilization ponds are most effective in warm climates. In colder climates, they can still be effective, but they require a longer retention time and thus a greater land area. In hot, arid climates, substantial water loss due to evaporation may occur in the dry season (e.g. approximately 25% of incoming volume in waste stabilization ponds in parts of Mexico [Jiménez, 2003] and Jordan [Duqqah, 2002]), and this will increase salinity of the effluent.

Waste stabilization ponds are most commonly the lowest-cost treatment option in tropical environments where inexpensive land is available (Arthur, 1983). They are relatively easy to operate and maintain, do not require skilled labour to operate and do not require electricity. However, the growth of vegetation in or near ponds must be controlled to prevent the creation of vector and snail intermediate host breeding habitats.

Wastewater storage and treatment reservoirs
Wastewater storage and treatment reservoirs (also called effluent storage reservoirs) have been used in several arid and semi-arid countries. They offer the advantage of storing wastewater until it can be used in the irrigation season, thus allowing the whole year's wastewater to be used for irrigation; a larger area of land is irrigated, and more crops are produced. The wastewater has to be pretreated (e.g. in an anaerobic pond) before it is added to the wastewater storage and treatment reservoir.

Procedures for designing waste storage and treatment reservoirs are detailed in Juanicó & Dor (1999) and Mara (2004). In general, if waste storage and treatment reservoirs are properly designed, operated and maintained, pathogen removals are very similar to those reported in waste stabilization ponds — i.e. a 2–4 log unit removal of viruses, a 3–6 log unit removal of bacterial pathogens, a 1–2 log unit removal of protozoan (oo)cysts and a 3 log unit removal of helminth eggs (if the waste storage and treatment reservoirs are operated as batch systems, helminth egg removal is 100%; Juanicó & Milstein, 2004).

Waste storage and treatment reservoirs also reduce evaporative losses and subsequent increases in salinity because of their greater depth (5–15 m) and smaller surface area. Whereas, as noted above, Jiménez (2003) found that a waste stabilization pond in an arid area of Mexico lost 25% of its inflow volume due to the high local rate of evaporation, Mara et al. (1997) reported that a waste storage and treatment reservoir in Brazil lost only 14% of its inflow volume during a four-month rest period during the hottest part of the year.

Constructed wetlands
Constructed wetlands are beds of aquatic macrophytes that grow in soil or, more commonly, sand or gravel. There are three main types: surface-flow, horizontal-flow subsurface and vertical-flow systems. Although, in principle, any aquatic macrophyte can be grown in constructed wetlands, the majority are planted with reeds and/or rushes; high-value ornamental flowers have also been grown successfully in constructed wetlands (Belmont et al., 2004). Constructed wetlands are secondary or tertiary treatment units; they are generally preceded by septic tanks, anaerobic ponds or conventional wastewater treatment plants. They are designed for biochemical oxygen demand (BOD), solids and nutrient removal, and not specifically for pathogen reduction. Nevertheless, some pathogen reduction does occur, although it may not be consistent. Reductions are <1–2 log units for viruses, <1–3 log units for bacteria, <1–3 log units for protozoan (oo)cysts and up to 3 log units for helminth eggs. Further details arc given in Rivera et al. (1995) and IWA Specialist Group (2000).

Constructed wetlands can be important sources of nuisance mosquitoes as well as, in some cases, mosquitoes of public health importance. Reports, among others, from the eastern seaboard of the United States of America, from southern Sweden and from Australia describe the phenomenon and present possible environmental management solutions (Schaefer et al., 2004; Victorian Government Department of Sustainability and Environment, 2004). Clearly, siting constructed wetlands at safe distances from human settlements is a measure of critical importance.

5.6.2 High-rate processes
High-rate processes are usually engineered systems built around complex infrastructure that have high flow rates and low hydraulic retention times. They usually include a primary treatment step to settle solids followed by a secondary treatment step to biodegrade organic substances, and they may include tertiary or advanced processes for the removal of specific contaminants.

These systems are often expensive, especially when tertiary treatment processes are required to meet microbial reduction targets. Additionally, most high-rate processes remove nitrogen, phosphorus and organic matter, which are all useful in irrigated agriculture.

In many (if not most) situations in developing countries, low-rate biological systems are more appropriate in terms of costs, pathogen reduction efficiency and simplicity of operation and maintenance.

Primary treatment
Primary treatment is achieved in sedimentation tanks with a retention time of approximately 2–6 h. Pathogen reduction is minimal, generally <1 log unit. However, where wastewaters have high numbers of helminth eggs, primary treatment can remove substantial numbers of eggs, even though the reduction is <1 log unit.

Chemically enhanced primary treatment
The pathogen reduction efficiency of primary treatment can be increased by incorporating coagulation/flocculation upstream and/or by using filtration downstream of gravity sedimentation (Metcalf & Eddy, Inc., 2003). Chemically enhanced primary treatment, also called advanced primary treatment, uses specific

chemicals (e.g. lime or ferric chloride, often with a high-molecular-mass anionic polymer) to facilitate particle coagulation and flocculation. Improving these processes increases the removal of suspended solids, including helminth eggs (Gambrill, 1990; Morrissey & Harleman, 1992; Jiménez & Chávez, 1998, 2002; Harleman & Murcott, 2001). Studies in Mexico City showed that advanced primary treatment was capable of producing effluents with 2–5 eggs per litre. When advanced primary treatment effluents were filtered through polishing sand filters, effluents with <1 egg per litre were produced at one third of the cost of a secondary treatment system (activated sludge), including sludge treatment and disposal 30 km away (Landa, Capella & Jiménez, 1997; Harleman & Murcott, 2001). Additionally, many virus particles are associated with particulate matter (suspended solids), and advanced primary treatment increases suspended solids removal from approximately 30% to 70–80% (Jiménez, 2003). Another advantage is that nitrogen, organic matter and phosphorus are only partially removed (Jimenez & Chavez, 1998, 2002).

Upflow anaerobic sludge blanket reactors
Upflow anaerobic sludge blanket reactors are high-rate anaerobic units used for the primary treatment of domestic wastewater. They have a hydraulic retention time of the order of 6–12 h (Mara, 2004). Wastewater is treated during its passage through a sludge layer (the sludge "blanket") by anaerobic bacteria. The treatment process is designed primarily for the removal of organic matter (BOD). However, upflow anaerobic sludge blanket reactors remove helminth eggs by 1–2 log units; upflow anaerobic sludge blanket reactor effluents in Brazil contain 3–10 eggs per litre (von Sperling et al., 2003; von Sperling, Bastos & Kato, 2004).

Secondary treatment
Secondary treatment systems, which follow primary treatment, are biological treatment processes coupled with solid/liquid separation. The biological processes are engineered to provide effective bio-oxidation of organic substrates dissolved or suspended in the wastewater. Secondary treatment processes comprise an aerobic microbial reactor followed by secondary sedimentation tanks to remove and concentrate the biomass produced from the conversion of wastewater organic constituents. The aerobic reactors use either suspended-growth processes (e.g. activated sludge, aerated lagoons, oxidation ditches) or fixed-film processes (trickling filters, rotating biological contactors). Although secondary treatment systems are designed primarily for the removal of BOD, suspended solids and often nutrients (nitrogen and phosphorus), they can, with optimized performance, reduce bacterial and viral pathogens by approximately 2 log units, protozoan (oo)cysts by 0–1 log unit and helminth eggs by approximately 2 log units, depending on the suspended solids concentration.

Tertiary treatment
Tertiary treatment refers to treatment processes downstream of secondary treatment, such as (a) additional solids removal by flocculation, coagulation and sedimentation and/or granular medium filtration; and (b) disinfection. When tertiary treatment processes are used, the overall sequence of wastewater treatment processes is generally described as "advanced wastewater treatment."

Coagulation, flocculation and sedimentation further reduce pathogens. Chemicals (e.g. ferric chloride, ferrous chloride, aluminium trisulfate, calcium oxide) are added to secondary effluents, which cause very small particles to combine or aggregate.

Larger aggregated particles then settle out of the liquid. Because viruses and bacteria are often associated with particulate matter, increasing its removal also increases their removal — for example, viruses can be reduced by 2–3 log units under optimal conditions (Jiménez, 2003); reductions for other pathogens are given in Table 5.2.

Filtration is also an effective additional step for removing pathogens. It can be used after primary treatment to improve helminth removal (e.g. after a coagulation/flocculation step in advanced primary treatment) or, more commonly, after secondary treatment. In filtration, pathogens and other particulate matter are removed by passing the effluents through sand or other porous media. There are several types of filtration, including high-rate granular filtration, slow sand filtration and dual-media filtration. Dual-media filtration uses two types of media with different properties to maximize the removal of particles with different properties. The effectiveness of filtration techniques for removing pathogens depends on the operating conditions. For example, high-rate and dual-media filtration are usually preceded by coagulation. By optimizing the coagulation process with dual-media filtration, bacterial reduction can increase from <1 log unit to 2–3 log units (WHO, 2004a). Efficient slow sand filtration requires optimum ripening, cleaning and refilling without short-circuiting (WHO, 2004a). Pathogen reductions achieved by filtration processes are given in Table 5.2.

The effectiveness of *disinfection* depends on several factors, including the type of disinfectant, contact time, temperature, pH, effluent quality and type of pathogen (WEF, 1996). Chlorine (free chlorine), ozone and ultraviolet irradiation are the principal disinfectants used to treat wastewater; chloramines may be used for advanced primary treatment effluents. Disinfection should be optimized for each type of disinfectant. In general, bacteria are the most susceptible to all three disinfectants. Helminth eggs and protozoan cysts/oocysts are the most resistant to chlorine and ozone, and certain viruses (e.g. adenoviruses) are the most resistant to ultraviolet disinfection (Rojas-Valencia et al., 2004). Although there are no data for helminth eggs, they are also expected to be resistant to ultraviolet irradiation. Pathogen reductions achieved by these disinfection processes are given in Table 5.2.

Effluents from activated sludge aeration tanks may be further treated by passage through *membranes*. The membranes have a very small pore size (20–500 nm), so they operate in the ultrafiltration and microfiltration range. They are thus able to achieve essentially complete reduction (i.e. >6 log units) of all pathogens, including viruses. However, membranes are very complex and expensive to operate (membrane fouling is a particular concern), although costs have been decreasing as the technology improves. A full description is given by Stephenson et al. (2000). Membranes provide an extremely efficient (but correspondingly expensive) combination of secondary and tertiary treatment.

5.7 Raw wastewater use

Globally, most wastewater used for crop irrigation is untreated, and often no other health promotion measures are in place to minimize the resulting adverse health impacts. As discussed in chapter 3, raw wastewater use in agriculture leads to a variety of health problems, especially helminth infections and diarrhoeal disease in both children and adults. A combination of the different health protection measures described in this chapter can be implemented to help make this practice safer. This section examines some practical steps that can be taken in the short and medium terms to reduce the adverse health impacts when raw wastewater is used for crop irrigation.

Crop restriction is the most suitable control measure when untreated wastewater is used for crop irrigation. Farmer education about the need for crop restriction is essential, especially concerning (a) the health risks to consumers if untreated wastewater were to be used for unrestricted irrigation and (b) which local "restricted" crops can be profitably grown. Local environmental health officers should regularly inspect the wastewater-irrigated fields to ensure that no unrestricted irrigation occurs.

Low-cost drip irrigation systems have been developed, and their use by farmers should be encouraged. They provide increased health protection and higher crop yields and use less water. Details are given by Polak et al. (1997), Kay (2001), Postel (2001), FAO (2002), Intermediate Technology Consultants (2003), von Westarp, Chieng & Schreier (2004) and International Development Enterprises (2005) (see also Table 4.3 and section 5.2). Simple wastewater pretreatment is required (section 5.6).

If untreated wastewater is used for unrestricted irrigation, then the 1–2 log unit pathogen reduction per day that occurs between the last irrigation and consumption is very important.

The simple food preparation measures detailed in section 5.4 should be actively promoted among local food handlers (in markets, in the home and in restaurants and food kiosks). A successful example of this is given by Faruqui, Niang & Redwood (2004), who reported results of a survey of produce consumers in Dakar, Senegal: this showed that approximately 70% were aware of the health risks from eating raw wastewater–irrigated vegetables, and they therefore either disinfected them or ate them only after cooking.

A survey of farmers who used raw wastewater for irrigation in Dakar, Senegal, revealed that less than half were aware of the health risks posed by the use of raw wastewater for irrigation purposes, and very few took precautions to reduce their exposure (e.g. by wearing gloves or shoes) (Faruqui, Niang & Redwood, 2004). Therefore, increasing awareness of the health risks may help to change behaviours.

Hygiene education and promotion are thus key public health interventions. Specific programmes and messages can be targeted at farmers, communities and produce consumers exposed either directly or indirectly to raw wastewater. Hygiene promotion can be conducted by local health assistants, on radio and television and through primary and secondary schools.

Other exposure control methods could include erecting low-cost fences around irrigation canals that transport raw wastewater and/or covering open sewers.

Immunization and chemotherapy are effective for preventing and reducing illness. Areas that rely on raw wastewater for irrigation should be targeted for immunization campaigns (especially typhoid, polio and hepatitis A). Regular mass chemotherapy campaigns against helminths in high-prevalence areas are also very effective (especially for 5- to 15-year-old children) and could be linked to hygiene promotion programmes for farmers and exposed communities. However, immunization and chemotherapy should not be seen as alternatives to wastewater treatment and other health protection measures. They are meant to be complementary health protection measures.

Untreated wastewater is commonly used for crop irrigation simply because the municipality has not constructed, or is unable to afford the construction of, a wastewater treatment plant. The health benefits of at least minimal wastewater treatment are potentially very large, however, especially if untreated wastewater is used for unrestricted irrigation. Crop restriction should be the first control measure applied (section 5.1). Simple wastewater treatment in anaerobic and facultative ponds (section 5.6.1) or advanced primary treatment with high-rate granular filtration (section 5.6.2) will usually achieve the health-based targets for restricted irrigation (Tables 4.1, 4.3 and 4.4). Helminth egg reduction is very important; if ≤1 egg per litre cannot be achieved, a reduction to ≤10 or ≤5 eggs per litre is a good initial step. Helminth eggs decrease in number in untreated wastewater over time, as even minimal wastewater treatment does much to decrease the prevalence of helminth infections by reducing the opportunity for reinfection, especially when regular mass chemotherapy campaigns are in force.

6

MONITORING AND SYSTEM ASSESSMENT

Monitoring has three different purposes: validation, or proving that the system is capable of meeting its design requirements; operational monitoring, which provides information regarding the functioning of individual components of the health protection measures; and verification, which usually takes place at the end of the process (e.g. treated wastewater, crop contamination) to ensure that the system is achieving its specified targets.

The most effective means of consistently ensuring the safety of wastewater use in agriculture is through the use of a comprehensive risk assessment and risk management approach that encompasses all steps in the process, from the generation and use of wastewater to the consumption of the product. This approach is captured in the Stockholm Framework. System assessment and its components are discussed in section 6.2.

The combination of health protection measures adopted in a particular wastewater use scheme requires regular monitoring to ensure that the system continues to function effectively. Monitoring, however, in the sense of observing, inspecting and collecting samples for analysis, is not sufficient on its own. Institutional arrangements must be established for the information collected in this way to provide feedback to those who implement the health protection measures. The responsibility for the monitoring of health protection measures should be clearly defined in the relevant legislation (see chapter 10).

6.1 Monitoring functions

The three functions of monitoring are each used for different purposes at different times. See Table 6.1 for a brief description of each type of monitoring. Validation is performed at the beginning when a new system is developed or when new processes are added and is used to test or prove that the system is capable of meeting the specified targets. Operational monitoring is used on a routine basis to indicate that processes are working as expected. Monitoring of this type relies on simple measurements (e.g. pH, turbidity) that can be read quickly so that decisions can be made in time to remedy a problem. Verification is used to show that the end product (e.g. treated wastewater, crop contamination) meets treatment targets (e.g. microbial quality specifications). Information from verification monitoring is collected periodically and thus would arrive too late to allow managers to make decisions to prevent a hazard break-through. However, verification monitoring can indicate trends over time (e.g. if the efficiency of a specific process was improving or decreasing). The validation and verification targets for effluents presented in the current guidelines are basically similar to what was referred to as recommended effluent standards or guidelines in the previous edition.

6.2 System assessment

The first step in developing a risk management system is to form a multidisciplinary team of experts with a thorough understanding of wastewater use in agriculture. Typically, such a team would include agriculture experts, engineers, water quality specialists, environmental health specialists, public health authorities and food safety experts. In most settings, the team would include members from several institutions, and there should be members from independent institutions, such as from universities.

Effective management of the wastewater use system requires a comprehensive understanding of the system, the range and magnitude of hazards that may be present and the magnitude of related risk levels, and the ability of existing processes and

Table 6.1 Definitions of monitoring functions

Function	Definition
Validation	Testing the system and its individual components to obtain evidence that it is capable of meeting the specified targets (i.e. microbial reduction targets). Should take place when a new system is developed or new processes are added.
Operational monitoring	The act of conducting a planned sequence of observations or measurements of control parameters to assess whether a control measure is operating within design specifications (e.g. turbidity following wastewater treatment). Emphasis is given to monitoring parameters that can be measured quickly and easily and that can indicate if a process is functioning properly. Operational monitoring data should help managers to make corrections that can prevent hazard break-through.
Verification	The application of methods, procedures, tests and other evaluations, in addition to those used in operational monitoring, to determine compliance with the system design parameters and/or whether the system meets specified requirements (e.g. microbial water quality testing for *E. coli* or helminth eggs, microbial or chemical analysis of irrigated crops).

infrastructure to manage actual or potential risks. It also requires an assessment of capabilities to meet targets. When a new system or an upgrade of an existing system is being planned, the first step in developing a risk management plan is the collection and evaluation of all available relevant information and consideration of what risks may arise during the entire production process. **Figure 6.**1 illustrates the development of a risk management plan.

The assessment and evaluation of a wastewater use system are enhanced through the development of a flow diagram. Such diagrams provide an overview description of the system, including the identification of sources of hazards, determining factors of associated risks and health protection measures. It is important that the representation of the wastewater use system be conceptually accurate. If the flow diagram is not correct, it is possible to overlook potential hazards that may be significant. To ensure accuracy, the flow diagram should be validated by visually checking it against features observed on the ground.

Data on the occurrence of hazards in the system combined with information concerning the effectiveness of existing controls enable an assessment of whether health-based targets can be achieved with the existing health protection measures. They also assist in identifying health protection measures that would reasonably be expected to achieve those targets if improvements are required.

To ensure accuracy of the assessment, it is essential that all elements of the wastewater use system are considered concurrently and that interactions and influences between elements and their overall effect are taken into consideration.

6.3 Validation

Validation is concerned with obtaining evidence on the performance of control measures, both individually and collectively. It should ensure that the system is capable of meeting the specified microbial reduction targets. Validation is used to test or prove design criteria. It should be conducted before a new risk management process is put into place (e.g. for wastewater treatment, wastewater application, produce washing/disinfection, etc.), when equipment is upgraded (e.g. new filter) or when new equipment or processes (e.g. addition of new coagulants) are added. It can also be used to test different combinations of processes to maximize process efficiency. Validation can be conducted at the facility scale or on a test scale. In a waste stabilization pond validation, for example, dye testing would be able to confirm that the design retention time was being achieved in practice.

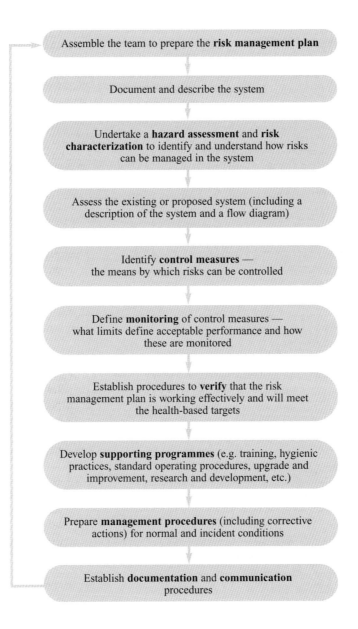

Figure 6.1
Development of a risk management plan (WHO, 2004a)

The first stage of validation is to consider data that already exist. These will include data from the scientific literature, trade associations, regulation and legislation departments and professional bodies, historical data and supplier knowledge. These data will inform the testing requirements. The second stage of validation is to conduct laboratory or pilot-level evaluations of the components and overall system under conditions that approximate those found at the actual site. A system should be validated for the different types of situations that occur (e.g. hot season vs cold season; dry season vs wet season; winter, spring, summer and autumn). Validation is not used for day-to-day management of wastewater treatment and use; as a result, parameters that may be inappropriate for operational monitoring can be used, and the lag time for return of results and additional costs from measurements can often be tolerated (WHO, 2004a).

6.4 Operational monitoring

Control measures are actions implemented in the system that prevent, reduce or eliminate contamination and are identified in system assessment. They include, for example, wastewater treatment and storage facilities, waste application techniques, use of protective clothing and sanitary conditions in the market or where the food is being prepared and consumed. If collectively operating properly, they would ensure that health-based targets are met.

Operational monitoring is the execution of planned observations or measurements to assess whether the control measures in a wastewater use system are operating properly. It is possible to set limits for control measures, monitor those limits and take corrective action in response to a detected deviation before the contamination passes through the system. Examples of limits are total suspended solids to indicate the level of particulate matter that might be associated with pathogens, turbidity, pH and flow rates. The presence or absence of plants in wastewater irrigation canals is an important indicator, since these may provide suitable habitats for disease vectors or snail intermediate hosts of schistosomes. Operational monitoring should take place around system parameters that indicate the potential for increased risk of hazard break-through. It is facilitated by simple measurements that can be taken quickly. For example, turbidity can be monitored quickly (often in real time) to indicate if a filter is malfunctioning or if a membrane is broken. Operational monitoring parameters are different for high-rate wastewater treatment and low-rate biological treatment systems. Examples of parameters that can be monitored are presented in Table 6.2.

The frequency of operational monitoring varies with the nature of the control measure; for example, checking physical infrastructure integrity (e.g. vegetation on the banks of wastewater treatment ponds) may occur monthly or less frequently, whereas monitoring turbidity in an activated sludge plant may be conducted in real time. If monitoring shows that a limit does not meet specifications, then there is the potential for a hazard break-through. The amount of time needed to correct an action should determine the rate of operational monitoring. For example, with waste stabilization pond systems, operational monitoring for various parameters (see Table 6.2) could take place at regular intervals of several weeks or longer, because the retention time is often long (e.g. 12–20 days). With wastewater treatment systems that have much shorter retention times (e.g. activated sludge), operational monitoring of parameters such as turbidity can take place online in real time.

A variety of physicochemical parameters should be monitored at regular intervals to verify the performance of a wastewater treatment system. Five-day BOD, chemical oxygen demand, total suspended solids, total dissolved solids, pH, temperature, exposure time and total nitrogen and phosphorus are examples of chemical parameters that are monitored for verification. Most of these parameters are monitored to prevent environmental impacts of wastewater discharge and to meet regulatory requirements for quality of wastes to be discharged. However, some may also be used as proxies for hazardous substances. For example, Jiménez & Chávez (1998) found a direct correlation between total suspended solids and intestinal helminth concentrations. It is easier to measure total suspended solids than to directly determine the concentration of helminth eggs, which requires a trained parasitology technician and suitable laboratory facilities.

In most cases, operational monitoring will be based on simple and rapid observations or tests, such as turbidity or structural integrity, rather than complex microbial or chemical tests. The complex tests are generally applied as part of validation and verification activities rather than as part of operational monitoring.

Monitoring needs to be conducted in such a way that it provides statistically meaningful information (e.g. sample duplicates), is directed at controlling the most important hazards and can inform changes to health protection measures. A monitoring programme should be designed in such a way that it can be performed within the technical and financial resources of any given situation. The objective is timely monitoring of control measures with a logically based sampling plan, to minimize negative public health impacts (WHO, 2004a).

6.5 Verification monitoring

Verification is the use of methods, procedures or tests in addition to those used in operational monitoring to determine if the performance of the wastewater/excreta use system is in compliance with the stated objectives outlined by the health-based targets and/or whether the system needs modification and revalidation.

For microbial reduction targets, verification is likely to include microbial analysis. In most cases, it will involve the analysis of faecal indicator microorganisms; in some circumstances, it may also include assessment of specific pathogen densities (e.g. helminth ova). Verification of the microbial quality of wastewater may be undertaken by local public health agencies.

Approaches to verification include testing of wastewater after treatment or wastewater at the point of application or use. Verification of the microbial quality of the wastes often includes testing for *E. coli* or thermotolerant coliforms. While *E. coli* is a useful indicator, it has limitations; the absence of *E. coli* will not necessarily indicate the absence of other pathogens. Under certain circumstances, it may be desirable to include more resistant microorganisms, such as *Ascaris* or bacteriophages (viruses that infect bacteria), as indicators for other microbial groups.

If wastewater is suspected to contain sizable industrial discharges, then periodic monitoring of the wastewater for heavy metals and chlorinated hydrocarbons may be warranted. Also, if crops with particular sensitivities (e.g. boron sensitivity) are being grown, then it will be important to monitor those chemicals that could have an impact on agricultural productivity (see Annex 2).

Table 6.2 Validation, operational monitoring and verification monitoring parameters for different control measures

Control measure	Validation requirements	Operational monitoring parameters	Verification monitoring parameters
Wastewater treatment	Effectiveness of treatment processes at inactivating/ removing pathogens and indicator organisms (*E. coli*, helminth eggs) System design (e.g. retention time, short-circuiting in waste stabilization pond by conducting dye testing) Analytical procedures for detecting indicators and/or pathogens (including measuring viability) Effectiveness of treatment in removing locally important toxic chemicals Analytical procedures and capabilities for detecting chemicals in wastewater, excreta or pond water	*Low-rate biological systems:* Flow rates BOD (loading rates may need to vary during colder periods) Algal concentrations and species types Dissolved oxygen at different pond depths (facultative and maturation ponds) *High-rate processes:* BOD Turbidity pH Organic carbon Particle counts Membrane integrity (pressure testing) Chlorine residual	*E. coli* Helminth eggs (including *Schistosome* spp., where appropriate) Locally important toxic chemicals
Health and hygiene promotion	Testing of promotional materials with relevant stakeholder groups	Local programmes in operation Promotional materials available Promotion included in school curriculum	Increased awareness of health and hygiene issues in key stakeholder groups Improved practices
Chemotherapy and immunization[a]	Effectiveness of different vaccines/drugs in preventing or treating locally important infections	Numbers of people vaccinated/treated Villages/schools targeted near wastewater use areas Frequency of campaigns	Reduced prevalence and intensity of infections Fewer disease outbreaks in targeted areas
Product restriction	Survey of product consumers to identify species always eaten after thorough cooking Analysis of marketability of different species/crops Economic viability of growing products not for human consumption	Types of crops grown in wastewater use areas	Water quality testing of wastewater to ensure that water used for unrestricted irrigation meets WHO microbial reduction targets

Table 6.2 (continued)

Control measure	Validation requirements	Operational monitoring parameters	Verification monitoring parameters
Waste application/ timing	Test the amount of time needed for pathogen die-off under different climatic conditions and for different pathogens/indicators between waste application and crop harvest to ensure minimal contamination	Monitor waste application timing and time to harvest	Analyse plant contamination
Produce washing, disinfection, cooking foods	Research on which methods are most effective in reducing contamination, pathogen inactivation Testing of educational materials among relevant stakeholders	Inspection by food safety authorities to ensure that proper procedures are being used at markets or restaurants where products are prepared	Periodic microbial testing of the hygiene of food preparation spaces in markets and restaurants, product testing to investigate where contamination occurs Inspection of markets to assess availability of safe drinking-water for product washing/freshening
Access control, use of personal protective equipment	Testing access control measures for effectiveness in preventing public exposures to wastewater Identifying which personal protective equipment is available at low cost that workers will wear Testing the effectiveness of the personal protective equipment in preventing exposure to hazards	Visual inspection of wastewater use areas for warning signs, fences, etc. Visual inspection of workers to ensure that they are wearing the appropriate personal protective clothing	Public health surveillance of workers to document reductions in skin diseases, schistosomiasis (where relevant) and hookworm
Intermediate host and vector control	Test system to evaluate its effect on insect vector breeding and/or survival and growth of relevant snail species Test control measures such as the reduction of emergent vegetation and its impact on the breeding of disease vectors or snail intermediate hosts Check for obstructed drains, seepage and a rise in groundwater levels that can result in pools of standing water	Visual inspection of facilities to observe vegetative growth in irrigation canals or treatment ponds Inspection of waters for relevant insect larvae or snail intermediate hosts	Public health surveillance to document vector-borne diseases or schistosomiasis in workers and local communities

[a] Chemotherapy and immunization are considered to be supplementary health protection measures and should not be used instead of other health protection measures such as wastewater treatment.

6.6 Small systems

Validation, operational monitoring and verification monitoring are important steps to identify and eventually mitigate public health issues that might be associated with wastewater use in agriculture. However, in some situations, the use of wastewater in agriculture can be difficult to monitor (e.g. in urban areas or in informal small-scale operations). Additionally, much of the wastewater use in agriculture that is practised is indirect and informal (e.g. irrigation with faecally contaminated surface waters) and thus harder to plan and control. Countries and local authorities may have limited budgets for validation and monitoring and thus will need to develop validation and monitoring programmes based on the most important local public health issues, the availability of professional staff and access to laboratory facilities.

When many small-scale wastewater irrigation operations exist, the national health or food safety authority may choose to validate health protection measures at a central research site and then disseminate information to relevant stakeholders (e.g. through the development of guidelines, through public health outreach workers, through agriculture extension workers or through local stakeholder workshops).

Operational monitoring should focus on visual inspections and safety audits without requiring difficult or expensive laboratory testing. For example, visual inspection of a facility will indicate the types of crops being grown or if workers are using boots and gloves. Similarly, food markets can be quickly inspected visually to detect unhygienic conditions or lack of safe water for product washing/freshening.

Verification monitoring may be easier to conduct at a central point (e.g. a wastewater discharge point or a market). Data from public health surveillance for faecal–oral diseases, schistosomiasis, intestinal helminth infections and other locally important diseases should be used to adjust health protection measures as necessary.

6.7 Other types of monitoring

6.7.1 Food inspection

Periodically, the microbial and chemical contamination of wastewater-irrigated crops should be tested. Products should be tested for *E. coli* or thermotolerant coliforms and helminth eggs where they are a hazard. The concentrations of heavy metals that may pose a health risk (e.g. cadmium, lead) should also be tested to ensure that they are within the safety limits specified by the Codex Alimentarius Commission.

6.7.2 Public health surveillance

Direct measurement of specific health outcomes (e.g. intestinal helminth infections, schistosomiasis and vector-borne diseases, such as filariasis) is possible and should be conducted periodically in exposed populations. This is discussed in the context of the Stockholm Framework in chapter 2.

7
SOCIOCULTURAL ASPECTS

Human behavioural patterns are a key determining factor in the transmission of excreta-related diseases. The social feasibility of changing certain behavioural patterns in order to introduce wastewater use schemes or to reduce disease transmission in existing schemes needs to be assessed on an individual project basis. Cultural beliefs vary so widely in different parts of the world that it is not possible to assume that any of the practices that have evolved in relation to wastewater use can be readily transferred elsewhere (Cross, 1985). However, there does appear to be a positive correlation between the occurrence of traditional waste use in societies and their population density, which has been called the "nutritional imperative." Societies that use excreta and wastewater or have used it in the recent past in agriculture or aquaculture are the most densely populated: Europe, India, China, Viet Nam and parts of Indonesia (Edwards, 1992).

Closely associated with cultural beliefs is the public perception of wastewater use. Even when projects are technically well planned and all of the relevant health protection measures have been included, the project can fail without adequately accounting for public perception. This chapter describes both of these aspects and how they relate to the use of wastewater in agriculture.

7.1 Cultural and religious beliefs

Untreated wastewater is currently used for agriculture in many parts of the world. Although there does not appear to be any significant sociocultural revulsion at this practice because of economic necessity, treated wastewater is much less objectionable in appearance than untreated wastewater and, from a socioaesthetic (as well as a health) perspective, is more suitable for agricultural use. Public fears may be allayed by suitably designed information programmes (see Box 7.1).

Box 7.1 Sociocultural acceptance of wastewater use in Nablus, West Bank and Gaza Strip, Palestinian Self-Rule Areas

During the development of a wastewater treatment and use demonstration plant in the town of Nablus, West Bank and Gaza Strip, Palestinian Self-Rule Areas, surveys of different stakeholders (i.e. general public, farmers and pilot project site visitors) were conducted. The majority of Palestinians are Muslims, and the surveys focused on sociocultural aspects of wastewater use. Conclusions from the survey were as follows:

- Villagers surveyed believed that the use of wastewater is acceptable in Islam providing that the effluent quality is safe and does not harm the health of the users.
- Drought and water shortage justified the use of wastewater in irrigation to conserve fresh water for other, more important purposes.
- Most of the people surveyed had never seen wastewater treatment plants.
- Most of the people surveyed thought that the use of raw wastewater was dangerous, whereas treated wastewater was an important resource.
- Survey respondents were willing to consume products grown with treated wastewater.
- Public perception and acceptance could be increased by exposing people to wastewater treatment demonstration plants and increasing public outreach efforts.

Source: Al Khateeb (2001).

In Islamic countries, it has been judged that wastewater can be used for irrigation provided that the impurities (*najassa*) present in raw wastewater are removed. According to Farooq & Ansari (1983), there are three ways in which impure water may be transformed into pure water:

1) self-purification of the water (e.g. removal of the impurities by sedimentation);
2) addition of pure water in sufficient quantity to dilute the impurities;
3) removal of the impurities by the passage of time or physical effects (e.g. sunlight and wind).

It is notable that the first and third of these transformations are essentially similar to those achieved by wastewater treatment processes.

In 1978, the Council of Leading Islamic Scholars of Saudi Arabia issued a fatwa (legal ruling on an issue of religious importance) concerning the use of wastewater in Islamic societies. The fatwa stated: "Impure wastewater can be considered as pure water and similar to the original pure water, if its treatment using advanced technical procedures is capable of removing its impurities with regard to taste, colour and smell, as witnessed by honest, specialized and knowledgeable experts. Then it can be used to remove body impurities and for purifying, even for drinking. If there are negative impacts from its direct use on the human health, then it is better to avoid its use, not because it is impure but to avoid harming the human beings." The Council of Leading Islamic Scholars prefers to avoid using wastewater for drinking (if possible) "to protect health and not to contradict with human habits" (Faruqui, Biswas & Bino, 2001).

Nevertheless, untreated wastewater is used in some Islamic countries, principally in areas where there is an extreme water shortage and then generally from a local wadi (ephemeral desert stream), but this is clearly a result of economic need and not of cultural preference.

In some Buddhist cultures, the use of wastewater and excreta as fertilizers in agriculture is in agreement with the central philosophy of reincarnation. It is not difficult to extend the philosophical concept of recycling human energy — birth, growth, decay, death and rebirth — to the harmonious concept of recycling earthly resources (Warner, 2000).

7.2 Public perception

The maintenance of good public relations, especially with respect to protection of consumer health, is a very important task. The public must have confidence that the food they are consuming is in no way injurious to their health. In this respect, programmes for the routine monitoring of wastewater and of produce quality are extremely important, as is the demonstrated absence of the transmission of infectious disease.

The public perception of wastewater use in agriculture varies much from one community to another. Where there is water scarcity or where wastewater is seen as a resource upon which people rely for their livelihoods, its use in agriculture is likely to be more acceptable. However, where people see it as a nuisance due to odour, perceived health or environmental impacts and lower property values, then it may be less acceptable.

It is important to recognize that even in situations where advanced wastewater treatment processes will be used to treat the wastewater and actual health risks will be very low, negative public perception can derail even well planned projects.

Bridgeman (2004) outlines several conclusions regarding public perception that arose during the development of various wastewater use projects in California, USA:

- Public perception varies by community; there is no one solution that will work in all communities. Outreach programmes must be based on a comprehensive understanding of the profile of the community that the planned project is to serve. From this, stakeholder-specific action plans should be developed.
- Community and stakeholder participation at the earliest stages of the project are important.
- The strength of public opinion regarding the use of wastewater should not be underestimated.
- A scheme will be approved by a community only following consistent, clear and reliable communication with that community. Key messages should be presented in a manner that is understandable to community members.
- Efforts to inform and involve the community should be proactive and not reactive.
- Successful projects require trust between the project planners and the potential recipients.
- Messages should focus on the positive benefits of the project.
- Education of the recipient communities is essential for projects to succeed.
- Timing of implementation and careful monitoring of public opinion are important. Communities may be more receptive to wastewater use projects when they are faced with a drought.
- Regardless of the economic and scientific basis behind the proposals for schemes, there may be people who, for their own reasons, will never accept the proposals.
- Monitoring programmes are key elements of projects to reassure the public.

7.2.1 Public acceptance of wastewater use schemes

To achieve general acceptance of wastewater use schemes, experience shows that active public involvement from the planning phase to the full implementation process is critical. Public involvement starts with the identification of and early contact with potential users, leading to the formation of an advisory committee and the holding of public hearings on potential use schemes. The exchange of information between authorities and public representatives ensures that the adoption of a specific water reuse programme will address real user needs and generally recognized community goals for health, safety, ecological concerns, programme cost, etc. (Crook et al., 1992; Helmer & Hespanhol, 1997).

Gaining public acceptance is easier once the need to use wastewater is established. If a community is aware of water scarcity and the need to conserve high-quality water sources for domestic purposes, they will be more willing to accept wastewater use. The use of wastewater becomes a solution to a problem instead of a problem in itself (UKWIR, 2005). As Figure 7.1 demonstrates, the public is more likely to accept wastewater use where there is a perception that there will be limited contact with the wastewater. Thus, using wastewater to irrigate fodder crops or crops that are always cooked before consumption is likely to be more acceptable to the public than using it to irrigate crops that will be eaten raw. As uses that increase the probability of coming into contact with the wastewater grow (e.g. using treated wastewater for laundry at the household level, storing treated wastewater in reservoirs used for recreation or as

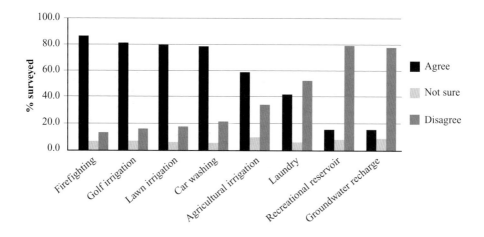

Figure 7.1
Attitudes towards wastewater use options (Robinson, Robinson & Hawkins, 2005)

drinking-water supplies or recharging groundwater used as drinking-water sources), the use of wastewater becomes less acceptable to the public.

Acceptance of wastewater use systems depends on the degree to which the responsible agencies succeed in providing the concerned public with a clear understanding of the complete programme; the knowledge of the quality of the treated wastewater and how it is to be used; confidence in the local management of the public utilities and on the application of locally accepted technology; assurance that the wastewater use application being considered will involve minimal health risks and minimal detrimental effects to the environment; and assurance, particularly for agricultural uses, of the sustainability of supply and suitability of the treated wastewater for the intended crops.

Figure 7.2 provides a flow chart for establishing programmes to involve the concerned community with all phases of wastewater use projects, from the planning phase to full implementation of the project, and Table 7.1 presents communication tools to address, educate and inform the public at different levels of involvement (Helmer & Hespanhol, 1997).

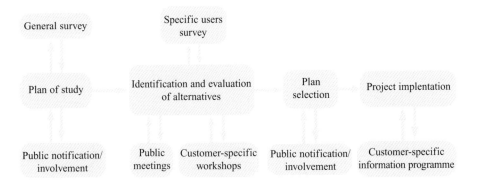

Figure 7.2
Developing a strategy for increasing public participation (adapted from Crook et al., 1992; Helmer & Hespanhol, 1997)

Table 7.1 Tools for increasing public participation in the decision to use wastewater

Purpose	Tools
Education and information	Newspaper articles, radio and television programmes, speeches and presentations, field trips, exhibits, information depositories, school programmes, films, brochures and newsletters, reports, letters, conferences
Review and reaction	Briefings, public meetings, public hearings, surveys and questionnaires, question and answer columns, advertised "hotlines" for telephone inquiries
Interaction dialogue	Workshops, special task forces, interviews, advisory boards, informal contacts, study group discussions, seminars

Source: Adapted from Crook et al. (1992).

8
ENVIRONMENTAL ASPECTS

T he use of wastewater in agriculture has the potential for both positive and negative environmental impacts. With careful planning and management, the use of wastewater in agriculture can be beneficial to the environment.

This chapter will present an overview of the beneficial and harmful components of wastewater and the impacts on soils and water bodies (surface water and groundwater). Suggestions for managing environmental impacts are also given.

Wastewater is an important source of water and nutrients for many farmers in arid and semi-arid climates. Sometimes it is the only water source available for agriculture. When wastewater use is well managed, it helps to recycle nutrients and water and therefore diminishes the cost of fertilizers or simply makes them accessible to farmers. This in itself has environmental consequences (e.g. less energy is needed to produce fertilizers [Sala & Serra, 2004], less phosphorus needs to be mined, etc.). Where wastewater treatment services are not provided, the use of wastewater in agriculture actually acts as a low-cost treatment method, taking advantage of the soil's capacity to naturally remove contamination. Therefore, the use of wastewater in irrigation helps to reduce downstream health and environmental impacts that would otherwise result if the wastewater were discharged directly into surface water bodies.

Nevertheless, agricultural wastewater use poses environmental risks. Possible effects and their relevance depend on each specific situation and how the wastewater is used. In many places, wastewater irrigation has arisen spontaneously and without planning — often the wastewater is untreated. In other situations, the use of wastewater in agriculture is strictly controlled. These practices will lead to different environmental impacts. Figure 8.1 shows schematically the generation and use of wastewater and how it interacts with the environment.

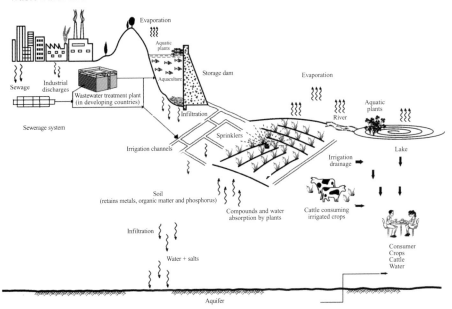

Figure 8.1
Simplified scheme of agricultural wastewater use and effects on the environment

The properties of domestic wastewater and industrial wastewater differ. Generally, the use of domestic wastewater for irrigation poses less risk to the environment than the use of industrial wastewaters, especially where industries use or produce highly toxic chemicals in their processes. Toxic chemicals from industrial processes are discharged into domestic wastewater in many countries, creating more serious environmental problems and endangering the health of the farmers and product consumers (see Box 8.1).

Box 8.1 Impact of industrial effluents on agriculture and aquaculture

The Bau Tram dam, located 10 km northwest of Danang City, Viet Nam, was built in 1961 with 1.2 million cubic metres of storage capacity. Water from the dam is used to irrigate 120 ha of rice paddies and produce fish. Irrigation water from the dam allows farmers to grow three rice crops per year (with a productivity of about 6 t/ha). Initially, the Bau Tram dam received the municipal wastewater of the local population. In 1990, however, the new industrial zone of Hoa Khanh began to divert 436 m^3/day of non-treated or barely treated industrial effluents into the reservoir. In some years, 50% of the agricultural production was lost, and aquaculture had to be stopped. In addition, water supplies were contaminated with heavy metals. Metals in the dam's sediments were transported to the fields during droughts and have contaminated the soils.

Source: Adapted from Raschid-Sally, van der Hoek & Ranawaka (2001).

8.1 Components of wastewater

The quality of wastewater (in terms of its physical and chemical characteristics) partly determines its environmental impacts. In arid and semi-arid areas, chemical concentrations are higher than in humid ones, because less water is used at the point of generation and higher evaporation rates during distribution and treatment reduce the water component. The following components of wastewater may have an impact on the environment:

- pathogens;
- salts;
- metals;
- toxic organic compounds;
- nutrients (nitrogen, phosphorus and potassium);
- organic matter;
- suspended solids;
- acids and bases (pH).

8.1.1 Pathogens

As indicated in chapters 2 and 3, wastewater may contain a variety of pathogens (i.e. bacteria, helminths, protozoa and viruses). These substances can contaminate crops, soil, surface water and groundwater. The survival of different pathogens in different media is described in chapters 2 and 3. From a health perspective, pathogens in the wastewater are generally considered to be the primary hazard, especially when inadequately treated or untreated wastewater is used in irrigation.

All of these types of pathogens can contaminate crops or soils. If wastewater is applied to extremely porous soils or thin or broken soils where groundwater is close to the surface (or is directly under the influence of surface waters), pathogens can contaminate aquifers. In general, the helminths and protozoa, because of their relatively large size, are removed more quickly in the top layers of soil through filtration. However, *Giardia* and *Cryptosporidium* have been detected in groundwater from a variety of different sites (Moulton-Hancock et al., 2000). Viruses and bacteria are smaller than helminths and protozoa and thus may be more mobile in the soil. Some viruses may be transported for long distances in aquifers, both vertically and horizontally (Yates & Gerba, 1998).

8.1.2 Salts

Perhaps the most important negative effect on the environment caused by agricultural wastewater use is the increase in soil salinity, which, if not controlled, can decrease productivity in the long term. Salinity is measured indirectly by a set of parameters such as conductivity, sodium adsorption ratio, sodium and chloride concentrations and dissolved solids. The rate at which soil salinity increases depends on the water quality and other factors, such as soil transmissivity, organic matter content, land drainage, irrigation rate and depth to the groundwater. For all these reasons, it is not easy to predict salinization rates, and it is more efficient to monitor salinity periodically at the site. There are four ways in which salinity affects soil productivity:

- It changes the osmotic pressure at the root zone due to high salt content.
- It provokes specific ion (sodium, boron or chloride) toxicity.
- It may interfere with plant uptake of essential nutrients (e.g. potassium and nitrate) due to antagonism with sodium, chloride and sulfates.
- It may destroy the soil structure by causing soil dispersion and clogging of pore spaces. This is exacerbated by both low-salinity waters and high sodium concentrations in the water in relation to calcium and magnesium concentrations in the soil. This is reflected in the sodium adsorption ratio (see Annex 1 for further discussion of the sodium adsorption ratio).

In the long term, wastewater use will always increase salinity of the soils and groundwater, because it contains more salts than fresh water. For that reason, it is necessary to combine the use of wastewater with practices to control salinization, such as soil washing, appropriate soil drainage and controlling salt inputs into the wastewater from detergents, water softeners, saline water infiltration, etc. (see Box 8.2). Salt content varies widely in municipal wastewaters, depending on the salinity content of the water supply and, to a lesser extent, saline discharges.

8.1.3 Heavy metals

The use of domestic wastewater for agriculture (treated or not) results in the accumulation of heavy metals in the arable soil layer (first soil layers used for cultivation after ploughing) without causing negative effects in crops, even if applied for long periods of time (several decades). The use of wastewater containing industrial discharges with high heavy metal concentrations leads to metal accumulation in soils and crops and has been associated with health problems in crop consumers (see chapter 3) (Chen, 1992; WHO, 1992; Yuan, 1993; Chang et al., 1995). Annex 2 contains a summary of studies on the impact of domestic and industrial wastewater irrigation on the concentrations of heavy metals in soils.

Regardless of the metal content of the wastewater, a metal will not be absorbed by plants unless it first reaches a threshold concentration in the soil (see chapter 4 for metal concentrations that pose a health risk; see Annex 1 for concentrations of heavy

---

Box 8.2 Salinization prevention in Israel

Israel uses 70% of its municipal wastewater for agricultural irrigation. This practice contributes to increasing salinity in soils and groundwater supplies, since treated wastewater has a higher salt concentration than fresh water. In Israel, salts in the wastewater come from detergents, water softening, hospitals, swimming pools, cleaning processes, meat processing and textile and dairy industries. Preventing the addition of salts to the wastewater at the point of generation is much cheaper than removing the salts once they have been added. An extensive control programme has been developed (see table below). Due to this programme and other measures, chlorides in sewage have dropped from 120 mg/l in 1992 to 60 mg/l in 2002; and boron from 0.6 mg/l in 1999 to 0.3 mg/l in 2002, with 0.2 mg/L predicted by 2008. Wastewater treatment processes that reduce the salt content (e.g. reverse osmosis) of the effluents have been adopted in the most sensitive environments.

Programme to control salt content in sewage

Date	Measure
1991	Requirement to use potassium salts instead of sodium in ion exchangers in certain industries
1993	Request to progressively discharge industrial softening brines to sea
1994	Regulation on quantity of salts used for ion exchanger regeneration
1995	Guidelines for controlling salt discharges from slaughterhouses
1996	Limitations on industrial brine discharges to sewer
1997	Standards on the proper construction and operation of evaporation ponds
1998	Complete prohibition of industrial discharges of brine to sewer
1999	Standard on the formulation of domestic and industrial detergents, progressively limiting the boron content from 8.4 g/kg to 0.5 g/kg in 2008, sodium from no limit to 4 g/kg for 2001 and chlorides from 61 g/kg to 40 g/kg for detergent for washing machines and from 121 to 90 g/kg for detergents for hand washing
2003	Public education on the use of salts in dishwashers and the use of detergents
2004	Limits on the concentration of salts in all industrial effluents: chlorides (430 mg/l), sodium (230 mg/l), fluorides (6 mg/l) and boron (1.5 mg/l)

Source: Adapted from Weber & Juanicó (2004).

---

metals that have an impact on agricultural productivity) and the metal is in a mobile phase (e.g. not adsorbed to soil particles or dissolved in soil water). Metals are bound to soils with pH above 6.5 and/or with high organic matter content. At pH levels below this value, organic matter is consumed or all feasible soil adsorption sites are saturated; metals become mobile and can be absorbed by crops and contaminate water bodies. Cadmium, copper, molybdenum, nickel and zinc are frequently present in wastewater and can be mobilized easily and absorbed by plants. Cadmium and nickel are more important health hazards than the other metals (see chapters 3 and 4) because of their greater toxicity to humans. Impacts of heavy metals on crops are complex, because there may be antagonistic interactions that affect their uptake by plants (Drakatos et al., 2002).

8.1.4 Toxic organic compounds

In wastewater, a great variety of toxic compounds may be present. Many are difficult to detect due to the lack of analytical techniques and the increasing number of compounds that are being produced and discharged to sewers. Domestic wastewater normally has low contents of toxic organic compounds, but concentrations can increase if it receives industrial discharges, agricultural runoff (i.e. containing pesticides and their residues), leaks from storage tanks or pipes (that contain products such as fuels), leachates from polluted soils, confinement sites and landfills and air pollutants deposited in rain. Among those compounds are industrial compounds (phthalates, biphenyl, *p*-nonylphenol, PCBs and tributyl tin), pesticides (atrazine, simazine, methoxychlor, 2,4-D, DDT, dieldrin, endosulphan and lindane), petroleum components, disinfection by-products or their precursors, hormones (from humans, such as 7-ethinylestradiol, or from plants, such as 17-α-estradiol, estriol) and pharmaceuticals (see below).

These pollutants may have carcinogenic, teratogenic and/or mutagenic effects. Additionally, some of them might interfere with hormone functions (endocrine disrupters) in animals or humans. If wastewater is treated prior to its use in agriculture, the concentration of many of these compounds will be reduced by adsorption, volatilization and biodegradation. Absorption of these substances by plants through roots is not likely to occur due to the large size and high molecular mass of many of these compounds, which reduces their mobility in soil and water (Pahren et al., 1979). It is possible that these chemicals can be transferred to the edible surfaces of crops irrigated with wastewater.

Endocrine disruptors may not degrade quickly in the environment. Mansell, Drewes & Rauch (2004) found that 17-α-estradiol, estriol and testosterone are not sensitive to photodegradation (i.e. less than 10% destruction after 24-h exposure to ultraviolet light). Thus, these compounds could remain on the surface of crops irrigated with wastewater. The concentrations of these compounds are usually extremely low, and to date only effects on animals in direct contact with polluted water have been demonstrated. Effects on humans have not been demonstrated.

USEPA (1981) concluded that, as long as irrigation is not performed continuously and at high rates, compounds such as endrin, methoxychlor, toxaphene, lindane, 2,4-D, 2,4,5-TP, silvex, tetrachloroethylene, *p*-dichlorobenzene and *o*-xylene are removed though soil infiltration. Synthetic organic compounds and organochlorides are adsorbed and biodegraded with time in soil. Cordy et al. (2003) studied the removal of 34 organic compounds that can be found in wastewater (some of them endocrine disruptors) and did not detect any of them after 3 m of infiltration through desert soils with a retention time of 21 days. Removal of endocrine disruptors such as steroidal hormones detected in treated and non-treated wastewater through infiltration in soils has also been demonstrated by Mansell, Drewes & Rauch (2004).

The dominant removal mechanism for these substances is adsorption. Removal efficiencies are greater in soils containing higher contents of silt, clay and organic matter. Additional attenuation, to below the detection limit, occurs by biodegradation, regardless of aerobic or anoxic conditions or the type of organic carbon matrix present (hydrophobic acids, hydrophilic carbon vs colloidal carbon).

A variety of pharmaceutical residues or their metabolic by-products in low concentrations can be detected in wastewater. This is a concern, because some of these chemicals retain their activity and, if they contaminate surface water or groundwater, could lead to human exposures through drinking-water. A number of biologically active pharmaceuticals and their metabolites have been identified in groundwater and drinking-water samples (Heberer, Reddersen & Mechlinski, 2002). The effects of these substances on the ecosystem and other animals are not yet known.

Studies with wastewater have shown that some of these substances may survive secondary and even tertiary treatments. A study of treated wastewater effluents (both secondary and tertiary treated effluents) that underwent further soil aquifer treatment indicated that most pharmaceuticals or their metabolic by-products were effectively removed by passage through the soil and after sufficient retention time in the aquifer. However, two drugs (carbamazepine and primidone) did not show significant reductions, even after six years of passage through the soil aquifer treatment system (Drewes, Heberer & Reddersen, 2002).

More research is needed to determine what chemicals are likely to persist in the environment, which of these may be harmful at the concentrations present in wastewater and what treatment techniques are most effective at removing them. Based on the soil aquifer study, it appears that chemicals with certain properties (e.g. acidic products or metabolites) are removed more easily than others (Drewes, Heberer & Reddersen, 2002).

8.1.5 Nutrients

As described in chapter 1, wastewater contains a variety of plant nutrients. Organic matter in the wastewater also can improve soil structure and fertility. A number of studies have demonstrated the positive impact of wastewater on crop productivity due to its nutrient content and organic matter (Day, Taher & Katterman, 1975; Day & Tucker, 1977; Bole & Bell, 1978; Marten, Larson & Clapp, 1980; Khouri, Kalbermatten & Bartone, 1994; Shahalam, Abuzahra & Jaradat, 1998; Parameswaran, 1999; Scott, Zarazua & Levine, 2000). Nitrogen, phosphorus and potassium are described below.

Nitrogen

Nitrogen is a necessary macronutrient for plants that can be found in wastewater as nitrate, ammonia, organic nitrogen and nitrite. The sum of all these forms is known as total nitrogen. Most plants absorb nitrates only, but normally the other forms are transformed into nitrates in the soil (National Research Council, 1996). Nevertheless, only 50% of the ammonia and 30% of organic nitrogen are assimilated by plants, since the rest is lost during transformation through several mechanisms, such as volatilization (Girovich, 1996). The main problem with nitrogen is that nitrates are very soluble in water, which is why, when irrigating crops, most of it is washed out. Often, this cannot be controlled, because many crops require large quantities of water to grow properly (Pescod, 1992). The quantity of nitrogen washed out depends mainly on the irrigation rate, the soil characteristics and the nitrogen content of the wastewater. Nitrogen needs to be added for each agricultural cycle, and nitrogen removed from the soils can affect other sites (e.g. if it enters groundwater or surface water). The amount of nitrogen that can be applied without leaching important quantities depends on the soil's nitrogen content (0.05–2%) and the crop demand, which oscillates between 50 and 350 kg of nitrogen per hectare, depending on the stage of the cropping cycle (Girovich, 1996). Nitrates are stable in groundwater and can build up to concentrations that might contribute to methaemoglobinaemia in bottle-fed infants if this water is used to prepare infant formulas (see chapter 3) (WHO, 2004a).

Phosphorus

Phosphorus is a plant macronutrient that is often scarce in soils in a form that is bioavailable to plants and almost always needs to be added with fertilizers. Phosphorus is relatively stable in soils and may accumulate in them, especially at or near the soil surface. Wastewater normally contains low amounts of phosphorus, so its use for irrigation is beneficial and does not negatively impact the environment (Girovich, 1996). This is the case even when wastewater effluents with high concentrations of phosphorus (e.g. effluents from dairy factories) are applied over long periods of time (Degens et al., 2000). However, because phosphorus builds up at the soil surface, it can affect surface waters through soil erosion and runoff.

It is predicted that accessible phosphate reserves will run out in 60–130 years (Steen & Agro, 1998). The mining of phosphate causes environmental damage, because it is often removed close to the surface in large open mines, leaving behind scarred land. Approximately 25% of the mined phosphorus ends up in aquatic environments or buried in landfills or other sinks (Tiessen, 1995). This causes eutrophication of water bodies, leading to more environmental damage. Moreover, to reduce eutrophication from phosphorus in wastewater discharged into surface waters, wastewater treatment plants require expensive, complex processes to remove it. Thus, the use of wastewater in agriculture recycles phosphorus, minimizes environmental impacts and reduces the costs of wastewater treatment to meet environmental regulations (EcoSanRes, 2005).

Potassium

Potassium is a macronutrient that is present in high concentrations in soils (3% of the lithosphere) but is not bioavailable, since it is bound to other compounds. Therefore, potassium needs to be added to soils through fertilizers. Approximately 185 kg of potassium per hectare is required. Wastewater contains low potassium concentrations, insufficient to cover the theoretical demand. The use of wastewater in agriculture does not normally cause negative environmental impacts associated with potassium (Mikkelsen & Camberato, 1995).

8.1.6 Organic matter

Wastewater not only adds nutrients to soils, but also enriches the humic content by adding organic matter that increases soil moisture, retains metals (through cationic exchange and the formation of organometallic compounds) and enhances microbial activity. This capacity to improve soils gives wastewater an additional advantage over synthetic fertilizers. The benefits observed depend on the original organic matter content in soils, which varies from <1.2% in poor soils to >5% in rich soils.

Most organic compounds of human, animal or plant origin contained in sewage are rapidly decomposed in soils. This has been extensively studied in soil aquifer treatment systems. Under aerobic conditions, breakdown is generally faster, more complete (into carbon dioxide, minerals and water) and performed with a greater variety of compounds than under anaerobic conditions. Stable, non-toxic organic compounds such as humic and fulvic acids are formed. Wastewater application in controlled conditions (i.e. through controlled irrigation rates and using intermittent flooding) allows the biodegradation of hundreds of kilograms of BOD per hectare per day, with no impact on the environment (Bouwer & Chaney, 1974). In cases where BOD concentrations are extremely high combined with high total dissolved solids levels, soil clogging can occur. However, this usually does not occur unless BOD levels exceed 500 mg/l (Darrell, 2002). In most cases, BOD levels are reduced to essentially zero after a short distance from the soil surface. However, at the end, water still contains some organic carbon, usually a few milligrams per litre due to humic and fulvic acids, but also possibly resulting from the presence of synthetic organic compounds. These recalcitrant compounds are not normally present in significant concentrations in municipal wastewater but can be important when industrial discharges are present. The behaviour of this kind of organic matter is described in section 8.1.4.

8.1.7 Suspended solids

Suspended solids in wastewater can clog the irrigating infrastructure, particularly if sprinklers and drip irrigation are used. In addition, if they are not biodegradable, they can also reduce percolation. Suspended solids from waste stabilization ponds may include algal particles, which add organic material and nutrients to the soil after they biodegrade.

8.1.8 Acids and bases (pH)

The pH of wastewater is usually slightly alkaline. When wastewater is combined with soil of adequate alkalinity, the acid/base soil equilibrium is not affected. Highly acid effluents (e.g. some industrial effluents) applied to soils with low alkalinity for long periods can modify pH. As mentioned in section 8.1.3, low pH values affect the mobility of heavy metals in the soil. Certain crops require specific pH ranges for optimum growth.

8.2 Environmental effects through the agricultural chain

The use of wastewater can affect soil or water resources through the agricultural chain, as shown in Table 8.1. on the following page. Some details concerning these impacts are given following Table 8.1.

8.2.1 Soils

Soil is a complex mixture of mineral and organic substances in concentrations that vary widely in different regions and climates. For this reason, it is very difficult to generalize as to which compounds are pollutants and in what concentrations. Effects depend not only on the physical and chemical properties of soils, but also on the type of crops, climate and quality and quantity of water used for irrigation. Najafi, Mousavi & Feizi (2003) indicate that even the irrigation method has an influence (for instance, metal accumulation is much lower when drip irrigation is used at 30 cm of depth than if it is performed at 15 cm or on the surface). The only relatively accurate methods to determine the effects on soils are:

- to measure the initial soil characteristics and monitor them over time; or
- to compare similar soils irrigated under similar conditions with either wastewater or fresh water.

The main and most common problem that wastewater use can cause in soils is salinization. This problem occurs even with fresh water if appropriate soil washing does not occur and land drainage is inadequate. The use of wastewater can accelerate the process of soil salinization due to its higher salt content. Salinization causes soil structure to collapse, losing pores and interconnections that allow water and air passage, and consequently:

- lateral drainage is increased;
- soils erode more easily;
- oxygenation is limited;
- root development is inhibited;
- plant growth is diminished or stopped.

Table 8.1 Effects on soils, crops and livestock, by type of compound

Parameter	Concentration in the irrigating water	Soil	Crops	Livestock
Nitrogen	Municipal wastewater with 20–85 mg TN/l	Acidification problems provoked by synthetic fertilizers are not observed	Increases productivity in quantity and quality	No problems reported
			Depending on soil's content and type of crops, problems can arise above 30 mg N-NO₃/l	
	Wastewater with >30 mg/l	No reported effects	Can increase succulence beyond desirable levels, causing lodging in grain crops and reducing sugar content in beets and cane	Forage, being the main food for cattle, can cause grass tetany, a disease related to an imbalance of nitrogen, potassium and magnesium in pasture grasses
			Beyond seasonal needs, may induce more vegetative than fruit growth and also delay ripening	
Phosphorus	Municipal wastewater with 6–20 mg/l	No reported effects	Increases productivity	
	Municipal wastewater with >20 mg/l	No reported effects	Reduce copper, iron and zinc availability in alkaline soils	
Potassium	Normal content in municipal wastewater[a]	No reported effects	Increases productivity	
	Content above normal municipal wastewater values[a]	No reported effects	Increases productivity	

Table 8.1 (continued)

Parameter	Concentration in the irrigating water	Soil	Crops	Livestock
Organic matter	Municipal wastewater with 110–400 mg BOD/l	Improves microbial activity and soil fertility Colloidal and suspended organic matter increase moisture and nutritious content, improving structure Diminishes salinity effects due to a higher water content Retains and binds heavy metals Depending on its composition and soil consumption, can release salts, nitrogen and metals	Increases productivity	No problems reported
	Content in wastewater greater than content in normal sewage[a]	Continuous irrigation and high organic matter contents may clog soil pores and favour an anaerobic population in the root zone Organic matter combined with nitrogen and continuous irrigation can cause important nitrogen losses by denitrification		
Salinity (variable, depending on the water supply content and type of discharges)	Wastewater with: TDS 250–850 mg/l Conductivity <3 dS/m SAR 5–9 Sodium <100 mg/l	No short-term effects observed Long-term salinization occurs at a rate that depends upon the frequency of soil washing and land drainage properties	Problems in sensitive crops with TDS of 450–2000 mg/l and conductivities of 0.7–3 dS/m Conductivities between 5 and 8 dS/m and non-sensitive crops do not display problems If soil is saline, crops absorb more salts, causing the crops' value to diminish in some countries and for some crops, such as vineyards	

Table 8.1 (*continued*)

Parameter	Concentration in the irrigating water	Soil	Crops	Livestock
Salinity (*continued*)	Wastewater with: TDS >2000 mg/l; Conductivity >3 dS/m; SAR >8; Sodium >100 mg/l	Loss of soil structure and capacity for water and air transport, and thus to sustain plants. Effects depend on conductivity and SAR values, frequency of soil washing and land drainage conditions	Impacts in almost all types of crops. Sodium diminishes yields in sensitive crops up to 100 mg/l. SAR >3 affects some crops, depending on the water conductivity. Productivity diminishes or even stops if salinization is very high	
Boron (very variable in wastewaters, depending on the water supply content and discharges)	Municipal wastewater with 0.7–3 mg/l; Municipal wastewater with >3 mg/l	No reported effects	Affects very sensitive (0.5–0.75 mg/l), sensitive (0.75–1 mg/l) and moderately sensitive (2–4 mg/l) crops. Affects moderately sensitive (2–4 mg/l), tolerant (4–6 mg/l) and very tolerant (6–15 mg/l) crops	
Chlorides	Wastewater with 30–100 mg/l; Wastewater with >140 mg/l	Can cause salinization, depending on other parameters as well as frequency of soil washing and land drainage conditions	Below 140 mg/l, no effects are observed. >140 mg/l, crops are affected, with very visible effects at concentrations >350 mg/l. Leaves of sensitive plants (crops and woody plants) are burnt when sprinklers are used for irrigation	
Alkalinity (carbonates and bicarbonates)	Wastewater with 50–200 mg CaCO$_3$/l; Wastewater with >500 mg CaCO$_3$/l	No reported effects. Concentrations above equilibrium conditions in soils precipitate calcium, affecting soil structure	In warm climates, bicarbonates burn leaves	No problems reported
Metals	Municipal wastewater or industrial effluents without high metal concentrations	Concentration in soil is increased with time in the first soil layers; depending on pH, organic matter content and irrigation time, metals are either bound to the soil particles or mobile	No effects are observed with normal metal contents of sewage	

Table 8.1 (continued)

Parameter	Concentration in the irrigating water	Soil	Crops	Livestock
Metals *(continued)*	Municipal wastewater or industrial discharges with high metals content	See Annex 2	See Annex 2	See Annex 2
	Aluminium and iron	Reduce phosphorus mobility	Can cause phosphorus deficiencies	
	Cadmium		Is toxic, and uptake can increase with time, depending on soil concentrations	May be harmful to animals in doses much lower than visibly affect plants
				Absorbed cadmium is stored in kidney and liver; remaining meat and milk products unaffected
	Copper			May be harmful to animals at concentrations too low to visibly affect plants
				Is not a health hazard to monogastric animals, but can be toxic to ruminants (cows and sheep)
				Tolerance to copper increases as available molybdenum increases
	Zinc and nickel		Cause visible adverse effects in plants before plant concentrations are high enough to be of concern in animals or humans	

Table 8.1 (continued)

Parameter	Concentration in the irrigating water	Soil	Crops	Livestock
Metals (continued)	Molybdenum			May be harmful to animals at concentrations that are too low to visibly affect plants
				Causes adverse effects in animals consuming forage with 10–20 mg/kg and low copper content
				Consumption of crops with more than 5 mg/kg is toxic to ruminants
				Molybdenum toxicity is related to the ingestion of copper and sulfate
Toxic organic compounds		Long term: some may biodegrade in soils	In general, their large sizes and high molecular mass do not allow them to be absorbed through plants	
		Some compounds, such as pesticides, might contain metals and contribute to their accumulation in soils	Can contaminate plant products through water contact during irrigation; sewage normally contains concentrations too low to cause problems	
Suspended solids	Municipal wastewater with 100–350 mg/l	Clog soils, depending on concentration, composition and soil porosity; >100 mg/l of mineral solids can cause problems		
		If soil is clogged, water infiltration rate diminishes and irrigation becomes less effective		
pH	Municipal wastewater with pH 7–7.4	No reported effects		

Table 8.1 (continued)

Parameter	Concentration in the irrigating water	Soil	Crops	Livestock
pH *(continued)*	Wastewater with pH out of the 6.5–8.5 range	If soil alkalinity is not sufficient to maintain pH above 6.5, metal solubilization can occur; when pH is maintained below 8.5, aluminium can be solubilized and soil deflocculated, and nitrogen can be lost by volatilization	Effects depend on the solubilized metal (see Annex 2)	

dS/m, deciSiemens per metre; SAR, soil adsorption ratio; TDS, total dissolved solids; TN, total nitrogen

Sources: NAS & NAE (1972); Seabrook (1975); Sidle, Hook & Kardos (1976); Benham-Blair & Affiliates, Inc. & Engineering Enterprises, Inc. (1979); Marten, Larson & Clapp (1980); Bouwer (1991); Metcalf & Eddy, Inc. (1991); Oron et al. (1992); Pescod (1992); National Research Council (1996); Siebe & Fischer (1996); Shahalam, Abuzahra & Jaradat (1998); Siebe (1998); ACTG (1999); Downs et al. (2000); Friedel et al. (2000); Simmons & Pongsakul (2002); AATSE (2004); Jiménez (2004); Jiménez, Siebe & Cifuentes (2004); Lee et al. (2004).

[a] Municipal wastewater content according to Metcalf & Eddy, Inc. (2003).

Salinity effects are, in general, mostly of concern in arid and semi-arid regions where accumulated salts are not flushed from the soil profile by natural precipitation and where the use of wastewater occurs. The risk of salinization, as already mentioned, is measured through a combination of parameters. A useful guideline is that, depending on the type of soils and the washing and drainage conditions, salinity problems can happen with conductivities >3 dS/m, dissolved solids >500 mg/l (being severe if >2000 mg/l) and a sodium adsorption ratio of 3–9 (see Annex 1 for more information) (Ayers & Wescot, 1985).

Sodicity, a specific kind of salinization, is produced by a high sodium ion concentration related to the concentrations of calcium and magnesium ions. This phenomenon can happen even with waters with low dissolved solid content and conductivity. Other compounds that can cause soil deflocculation are carbonates and bicarbonates. The effect is moderate between bicarbonate concentrations of 90 and 500 mg/l; above 500 mg/l, problems can arise. Wastewater is not the only factor that causes salinization; inefficient soil and subsoil drainage, climate and the type of soil also can cause it, even with freshwater irrigation.

Changing the quality of the irrigation water can also affect soils, since a new equilibrium must be reached. For instance, if water with an elevated organic content is replaced by another one with reduced organic content, two effects can be observed (Siebe & Fischer, 1996):

1) salinization problems due to an increase in salt concentrations near the roots as moisture is lost;
2) metal mobilization, since there is no organic matter to bind them.

The greater the differences in the water quality between the original water and the new water source, the more noticeable the effects on the soil.

Soil has a tremendous capacity to adsorb heavy metals (see Annex 1) — so much so that it has been estimated that domestic wastewater of average metal concentration (values can be consulted in Metcalf & Eddy, Inc., 2003) could be applied to the land for several hundred years without fully exhausting the capacity of the soil to adsorb heavy metals (Reed, Thomas & Kowal, 1980). Metals are retained in the upper layers, remaining bound to the organic fraction or precipitated due to pH. Only a small fraction of metals is infiltrated to lower layers, and a still much smaller fraction is absorbed by crops. For instance, around 80–94% of cadmium, copper, nickel and zinc are removed in the first 5–15 cm of soil, 5–15% runs off and 1–8% is absorbed by grasses (Peters, Lee & Bates, 1980).

8.2.2 Groundwater

Table 8.2 describes the impacts some of the substances found in wastewater can have on groundwater and surface water. An indirect consequence of irrigated agriculture with either fresh water or wastewater is aquifer recharge (Table 8.3; Box 8.3). Recharge of aquifers is almost always unplanned and has the advantage of increasing the local availability of water. This should be considered when wastewater irrigation schemes are being planned.

Table 8.2 Impact on groundwater and surface water bodies by different compounds during irrigation with wastewater

Compound	Impact	Relative impact on groundwater or surface water	
		Groundwater	Surface water
Nitrogen	May contaminate underground and surface water bodies by infiltration and irrigation runoff. The amount of nitrogen leached depends on crop demand, hydraulic load due to rain and irrigation water, soil permeability and nitrogen content in soils.	High	Medium
Phosphorus	Agricultural runoff containing phosphorus can cause the growth of aquatic plants as a result of eutrophication in surface water bodies (reservoirs and lakes), which can lead to the obstruction of irrigation infrastructure (filters, weirs, pipes and spillways) and clog filters in water treatment plants.	Not significant	Medium
Biodegradable organic matter	If runoff contains high levels of organic matter, the organic matter can consume dissolved oxygen in lakes and rivers.	Not significant	Medium
Salinity	Saline soil leachates contaminate surface and underground water bodies; up to a certain level, it can limit water use.	Medium	Low
	TDS > 500 mg/l causes flavour but not health problems in water supplies.		
	Very high concentrations have laxative effects on consumers and corrode water distribution equipment.		
Boron	Boron from wastewater is not removed by treatment, almost not retained in soils and not absorbed by plants.	Medium	Low
	Although it is an essential element, it easily becomes toxic above the required levels.		
	By leaching, it enters groundwater and, through runoff or from polluted aquifers, surface water bodies.		
	Accumulation in water bodies limits their use, mainly for irrigation.		
	Some crops are sensitive to boron (see Annex 1).		
Heavy metals	By leaching from acid soils, they can reach aquifers and enter surface waters through runoff.	Low	Low
Toxic organic compounds	Mostly removed by soils.	Not significant	Not significant

TDS, total dissolved solids

Table 8.3 Aquifer recharge during wastewater use in agriculture

Effect	References
After 35 years of irrigation with domestic wastewater in Haroonabad, Pakistan, groundwater quality beyond the site has been modified compared with a similar zone irrigated with fresh water as follows: salinity 5.4 ± 2 vs 2.8 ± 0.4 dS/m, *E. coli* 338 vs 20 MPN/100 ml and nitrates 68 vs 47 mg NO_3/l	Matsuno et al. (2004)
In Gabal, the Asfar farm in the Greater Cairo region, untreated or primary-treated wastewater used for irrigation since 1915 has led to reduced salinity of groundwater (the aquifer was saline to begin with) as well as its recharge.	Farid et al. (1993); Rashed et al. (1995)
In Mezquital, Mexico, more than 25 m³/s of wastewater are infiltrated to the aquifer as a consequence of agricultural irrigation. The irrigating water improves its quality through its storage in reservoirs and passage through channels and soils. The aquifer provides a water supply for more than 300 000 people, even though salinity is increasing.	BGS-CNA (1998); Jiménez, Siebe & Cifuentes (2004)

MPN, most probable number

Water application in excess of plant needs and the soil retention capacity leads to water infiltration, which also occurs during storage and transportation prior to use. Foster et al. (2004) analysed aquifer recharge from wastewater irrigation in Miraflores, the periurban area of Lima, Peru, Wagi Dhuleil, Jordan, Mezquital Valley, Mexico, Leon, Mexico, and Hat Yai, Thailand, and estimated infiltration of at least 1000 mm/year, a value that in many cases exceeds the local pluvial precipitation. Rashed et al. (1995) estimated that infiltration equals 50–70% of the water used for agriculture.

The impact on groundwater quality depends on several factors, such as the irrigation rate, the irrigation water quality, the treatment given to water by soils, the vulnerability of the aquifer, the form in which irrigation is performed, the rate of the artificial recharge compared with the natural rate, the original quality of underground water and its potential use, the time under irrigation and the type of crops (Foster et al., 2004).

Aquifers beneath agricultural fields often display high nitrate concentrations, because both the use of wastewater and artificial fertilizers add nitrogen to soils faster than plants can absorb it, and hence nitrogen is removed by water as any other salt would be. Nitrates are also stable in groundwater and thus can increase in concentration over time.

In the long term, salinity in aquifers generally increases. Based on the original quality, the present and future use and the interconnections between the aquifer and other water bodies, this effect may or may not be important (Farid et al., 1993). If the groundwater depth is less than 1–1.5 m, there are severe risks of increasing soil salinity; thus, it is frequently suggested that the use of wastewater for irrigation should be restricted to areas with groundwater depths greater than 1.5–3 m.

Normally, metals have little impact on aquifers, since domestic wastewater contains low levels. According to Leach, Enfield & Harlin (1980) and USEPA (1981), the metals that are most toxic to humans — cadmium, lead and mercury — were absent in groundwater at five sites in the United States of America after 30–40 years of applying secondary and primary effluents at rates between 0.8 and 8.6 m/year for different crops. The reason given was that soil pH was above 6.5, and metals were bound tightly by soil particles.

Box 8.3 Wastewater irrigation and aquifer recharge in the Mezquital Valley in Tula, Mexico

Water balance in Mexico City and the Mezquital Valley

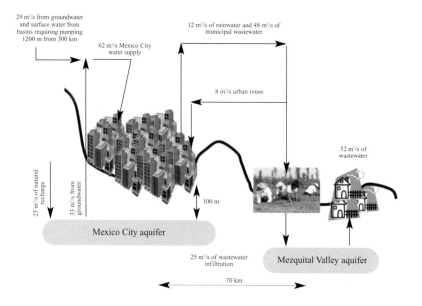

Figure 8.2
Aquifer recharge in the Mezquital Valley resulting from wastewater irrigation

Near Mexico City, in the Mezquital Valley, 85 000 ha are irrigated with mostly untreated wastewater from the city. Wastewater is appreciated by Mezquital farmers, since it allows agricultural development in an area with 550 mm annual precipitation and soils with low organic matter content that require irrigation and fertilizers to be productive. In fact, farmers are against wastewater treatment that could remove "the substance" — that is, the fertilizing materials. Wastewater contributes 2400 kg of organic matter, 195 kg of nitrogen and 81 kg of phosphorus to the soils per hectare each year. After 80 years of irrigation, phosphorus in the soils has increased from 6 to 20 g/m^2, nitrogen from 0.2 to 0.8 kg/m^2 and organic matter from 2% to 5%. Metals in the soils have also increased, from three to six times their original values.

It has been observed that wastewater application increases microbial activity and soil denitrification capacity. However, salinity has increased and has reduced microbial activity in sites with more than 65 years of irrigation. Salinity is becoming a problem in zones with poor soil drainage (vertisol soils) located in the lower parts of the valley (Friedel et al., 2000). Crops grown at sites with more than 80–100 years of irrigation do not show elevated metal concentrations. Metals are fixed to soils by pH and organic matter content. However, salinity in crops has increased (e.g. in alfalfa, from 1.5 to 4 g/kg in sites watered for more than 80 years) (Siebe, 1998).

Due to the high irrigation rate (1.5–2.2 m/year) and to the storage and transport of wastewater in unlined dams and channels, the aquifer is being recharged, and new underground deposits have been formed. In 1998, the British Geological Survey calculated that the water infiltration rate was at least 25 m^3/s. This incidental recharge

Box 8.3 (continued)

has happened in such magnitude and for such a long time that the phreatic level has risen in some places from 50 m deep to the surface. Springs have appeared with flows between 40 and 600 l/s. These springs have become the only water supply for more than 300 000 people. Fortunately, the transport of wastewater in channels and its use in irrigation have improved its quality. By the time the water enters the aquifer, organic matter has been reduced by 95%, metal concentrations by 70–90%, microorganisms by >99.9% and levels of more than 130 organic compounds by >99%. Pollutant removal is different for each compound, depending on its trajectory through the Valley, its passage rate through soil and the type of removal mechanisms involved. Salt concentrations (i.e. dissolved solids, conductivity or nitrates) have increased.

The new water deposits in the Mezquital Valley have created ecological change; from being a semi-arid zone, now the area has several springs and wetlands with a variety of animals and plants (including "acociles," a type of Mexican shrimp that grows only in very clean waters). Owing to the increasing demand for fresh water in Mexico City, where there is a water deficit of 5 m^3/s, the government is considering returning 6–10 m^3/s from the water accumulated in the Mezquital Valley subsoil. This is an attractive option compared with others that require importing water from sites located more than 1000 m lower than Mexico City and 200 km away ("The Mezquital" is only 150 m lower and 100 km away) or from sites closer to Mexico City but whose population does not want its water to be taken away, or treating Mexico City's wastewater to inject it into the aquifer for human consumption, thus seriously decreasing its current use in the Mezquital Valley.

Sources: Jiménez & Chávez (2004); Jiménez, Siebe & Cifuentes (2004).

Organic matter reaching aquifers from percolating treated wastewater varies in concentration between 1 and 5 mg of total organic carbon (TOC) per litre. If untreated wastewater is used, the content can rise to 6–9 mg of TOC per litre (Foster et al., 2004). Both ranges are higher than what is commonly accepted as safe for recharge of human drinking-water sources (1–2 mg of TOC per litre); even for low concentrations, the concern would be what kind of compounds are part of the TOC. High TOC can lead to the formation of disinfection by-products if water is treated for human consumption and disinfected with chlorine (see WHO, 2004a, for more discussion of disinfection by-products). There may also be toxic compounds of industrial origin or possibly endocrine disrupters. Fortunately, absorption of these types of substances is very effective in soils, as described in section 8.1.4.

In order to avoid the negative effects on the environment of using wastewater for agriculture due to its infiltration, it is recommended to (Foster et al., 2004):

- improve agricultural irrigation practices;
- establish criteria to operate wells used to supply water for human consumption in the surroundings (establish safe distances to the irrigation site, depth of extraction and appropriate construction);
- promote wastewater use for agriculture, preferably in zones where aquifers are less vulnerable;
- routinely monitor groundwater.

8.2.3 Surface water
Surface water bodies are affected by wastewater use in agriculture because they receive water from drainage and runoff; although the impact is lower than that from direct discharge of wastewater to them, effects also occur. Impacts depend on the type of water body (rivers, irrigation channels, lakes or dams) and their use, as well as the hydraulic retention time and the function played within the ecosystem. The main

impact arises from pathogen contamination of surface water bodies, which might lead to health impacts for downstream users through drinking-water, recreational water contact or contaminated food sources (e.g. shellfish, or crops contaminated when the water source is used for irrigation downstream).

If high amounts of biodegradable organic matter enter surface waters, it can deplete dissolved oxygen, thus impacting aquatic organisms and causing an odour nuisance. If too much nitrogen or phosphorus is washed into water bodies, it can lead to eutrophication and subsequent oxygen depletion, which also harms aquatic plant and animal life and may impair the aesthetic value of the water body. There is also evidence that nutrient enrichment of water bodies may facilitate the growth of algae that produce harmful toxins (Chorus & Bartram, 1999).

Evidence suggests that toxic organic chemicals associated with wastewater will only minimally impact surface water bodies due to their adsorption to soil particles after application.

8.3 Management strategies for reducing environmental impacts

In Tables 8.4 and 8.5, recommendations to control some of the impacts described are presented by polluting agent or problem. Many of the management approaches also conform to good agricultural practices, which are discussed in Annex 1. Management strategies might vary during the course of the growing season. For example, nitrogen concentrations in the wastewater should be matched to the needs of the crops. As crops develop, the amount of nitrogen they need and/or can absorb changes. In some crops (e.g. rice or tomatoes), application of too much nitrogen will cause excessive vegetative growth, diminishing the quality of edible portions. Some of the management strategies involve upstream interventions to reduce salt inputs or the addition of toxic chemicals (both organic substances and heavy metals) from industrial discharges.

Table 8.4 Control measures by polluting agent

Compound	Control measure
Nitrogen in excess	Dilute wastewater with fresh water when possible
	Limit the quantity of wastewater applied
	Remove excess nitrogen from wastewater
Organic matter	Do not continuously apply wastewater, to allow soil to biodegrade it
	Enhance removal of organic matter from wastewater
Salinity	Avoid the use of water with 500–2000 mg TDS/l or 0.8–2.3 dS/m electrical conductivity, depending on the type of soil and land drainage
	Reduce upstream salt use and discharge into wastewater
Chlorides	With sprinklers, only use water with <100 mg/l
	In irrigation by flooding, use water with <350 mg/l
	Irrigate by night to prevent leaf burn
Toxic organic compounds in soil and crops	Pretreat or segregate industrial discharges from sewage
	Promote cleaner production in industries, to avoid using toxic compounds
	Educate society to use less toxic compounds and, when used, dispose of them safely
Metals	Pretreat or segregate industrial discharges from sewage
	Use wastewater only in soils having a pH >6.5
Suspended solids	Use water without solids >2–5 mm
	Remove suspended solids by pretreatment of wastewater
	Plough soils when clogged

TDS, total dissolved solids
Sources: Seabrook (1975); Bole & Bell (1978); Reed, Thomas & Kowal (1980); USEPA (1981); Ayers & Wescot (1985); Phene & Ruskin (1989); Bouwer (1991); Oron et al. (1991, 1992); Pescod (1992); Farid et al. (1993); Chang et al. (1995); National Research Council (1996); Jiménez & Chávez (1997); Strauss (2000); Cornish & Lawrence (2001); AATSE (2004); Ensink, Simmons & van der Hoek (2004); Ensink et al. (2004); Foster et al. (2004).

Table 8.5 Control measures according to the kind of problem

Problem	Control measure
Evaporation and infiltration of water during storage	Use compact lagoons in series lined with impermeable materials (clay, plastic) to prevent loss of water to evaporation and infiltration
Clogging of irrigation systems	Use water with low total suspended solids content
	Use irrigation methods not affected by solids
Sprinkler clogging/corrosion	Clogging and corrosion can be controlled by using water with <100 mg of chlorine per litre, <70 mg of sodium per litre and <1.5 mg of iron and manganese per litre
Soil salinity and sodicity	Increase soil washing, improve ground drainage and/or apply soil amenders
	Dilute water with sodium adsorption ratio >8 and electrical conductivity >2.3 dS/m
Formation of a biological soil layer that blocks water infiltration	Reduce the quantity of water applied and/or increase flood and dry periods
Infiltration to subsoil of low-quality water	Irrigate in places where aquifer level is >3 m below the surface and soil permeability is 60–2000 mm/day
	Reduce the hydraulic load

Table 8.5 (continued)

Problem	Control measure
Joint leaching of nitrogen and organic matter	Promote biological denitrificaction in soil by creating an appropriate carbon to nitrogen ratio, promoting anaerobic conditions in soils and avoiding salt accumulations that inhibit denitrification bacteria
Contamination of water bodies	Adapt irrigation rates according to crop demands and allow sufficient passage of water through soil
	Irrigate in sites located 500–1000 m from surface water bodies or more than 3 m from aquifers used as water supply
Water pollution with pesticides	Do not irrigate immediately after pesticide application
	Do not over-apply pesticides
	Use integrated pest management approaches to reduce pesticide use

9

ECONOMIC AND FINANCIAL CONSIDERATIONS

conomic factors are especially important when studying and appraising the feasibility of a new scheme for the use of wastewater. Even an economically worthwhile project can fail, however, without careful financial planning.

Economic analysis and financial considerations are crucial for encouraging the safe use of wastewater. Economic analysis seeks to establish the economic feasibility of a project and enables comparisons between different options. The (often hidden) cost transfers to other sectors (e.g. the health and environmental impacts on downstream communities) need to be included in a cost analysis. This can be facilitated by the use of the multiple-objective decision-making process.

Financial planning looks at how the project is to be paid for. In establishing the financial feasibility of a project, it is important to determine the sources of revenues and clarify who will pay for what. The ability to profitably sell products grown with wastewater or to sell the treated wastewater themselves also needs analysis. Section 9.3 discusses the assessment of market feasibility.

9.1 Economic feasibility

Economic analyses seek to establish whether a project is affordable and has a positive internal rate of return. There are different methods that can be used to analyse a project and its implementation at the macroeconomic level.

9.1.1 Cost–benefit analysis

Within the framework of a cost–benefit analysis, monetary values are assigned to all expected costs and benefits of the project whenever possible to determine the feasibility of the project in relation to the economy of the country. The economic analysis of a wastewater use project is undertaken to determine the benefits emanating from a project in relation to the economic resources invested in it. It informs a decision as to whether it is worthwhile to proceed with it (Squire & Van Der Tak, 1975; Gittinger, 1982). This requires a calculation of the marginal costs and benefits of the project — that is, the differences between the costs and benefits of the project and the costs and benefits of the alternative. For a scheme to be economically viable, its marginal benefits should exceed its marginal costs. Traditionally, the health sector has used cost-effectiveness analyses for economic evaluations of different options for health interventions, but recently the advent of the DALY has facilitated a shift towards cost–benefit analysis, greatly improving the communications with other sectors on economic issues.

When used to analyse wastewater use schemes, cost–benefit analyses have the advantage of producing comparable data for a range of different options, which can be used for decision-making. As part of the overall costs, appraisals should therefore explicitly include not only those of the system hardware but also those for other components, such as planning and administration, hygiene promotion campaigns and the health and environmental impacts on downstream communities associated with different options. For a given situation, planners should consider the costs of implementing different combinations of health protection measures, as presented in Figure 4.1. Table 9.1 presents information on the costs of different wastewater treatment systems. Costs are meant to be illustrative, as they will vary significantly from location to location.

Table 9.1 Economic considerations for different wastewater treatment systems

System	Land requirements (m²/inhabitant)	Power for aeration		Sludge volume		Costs	
		Installed power (W/inhabitant)	Consumed power (kWh/inhabitant per year)	Liquid sludge to be treated (litres per inhabitant per year)	Dewatered sludge to be disposed of (litres per inhabitant per year)	Construction (US$/inhabitant)	Operation and maintenance (US$/inhabitant per year)
Primary treatment (septic tanks)	0.03–0.05	0	0	110–360	15–35	12–20	0.5–1.0
Conventional primary treatment	0.02–0.04	0	0	330–730	15–40	12–20	0.5–1.0
Advanced primary treatment (chemically enhanced)	0.04–0.06	0	0	730–2500	40–110	15–25	3.0–6.0
Facultative pond	2.0–4.0	0	0	35–90	15–30	15–30	0.8–1.5
Anaerobic pond + facultative pond	1.2–3.0	0	0	55–160	20–60	12–30	0.8–1.5
Facultative aerated lagoon	0.25–0.5	1.2–2.0	11–18	30–220	7–30	20–35	2.0–3.5
Complete-mix aerated lagoon + sedimentation pond	0.2–0.4	1.8–2.5	16–22	55–360	10–35	20–35	2.0–3.5
Anaerobic pond + facultative pond + maturation pond	3.0–5.0	0	0	55–160	20–60	20–40	1.0–2.0
Anaerobic pond + facultative pond + high-rate pond	2.0–3.5	<0.3	<2	55–160	20–60	20–35	1.5–2.5
Anaerobic pond + facultative pond + algae removal	1.7–3.2	0	0	60–190	25–70	20–35	1.5–2.5
Slow-rate treatment	10–50	0	0	–	–	8–25	0.4–1.2
Rapid infiltration	1.0–6.0	0	0	–	–	12–30	0.5–1.5
Overland flow	2.0–3.5	0	0	–	–	15–30	0.8–1.5
Constructed wetlands	3.0–5.0	0	0	–	–	20–30	1.0–1.5
Septic tank + anaerobic filter	0.2–0.35	0	0	180–1000	25–50	30–50	2.5–4.0
Septic tank + infiltration	1.0–1.5	0	0	110–360	15–35	25–40	1.2–2.0

Table 9.1 (continued)

System	Land requirements (m²/inhabitant)	Power for aeration		Sludge volume		Costs	
		Installed power (W/inhabitant)	Consumed power (kWh/inhabitant per year)	Liquid sludge to be treated (litres per inhabitant per year)	Dewatered sludge to be disposed of (litres per inhabitant per year)	Construction (US$/inhabitant)	Operation and maintenance (US$/inhabitant per year)
UASB reactor	0.03–0.10	0	0	70–220	10–35	12–20	1.0–1.5
UASB + activated sludge	0.08–0.2	1.8–3.5	14–20	180–400	15–60	30–45	2.5–5.0
UASB + high-rate trickling filter	0.1–0.2	0	0	180–400	15–55	25–35	2.0–3.0
UASB + maturation ponds	1.5–2.5	0	0	150–250	10–35	15–30	1.8–3.0
UASB + facultative aerated pond	0.15–0.3	0.3–0.6	2–5	150–300	15–50	15–35	2.0–3.5
UASB + overland flow	1.5–3.0	0	0	70–220	10–35	20–35	2.0–3.0
Conventional activated sludge	0.12–0.25	2.5–4.5	18–26	1100–3000	35–90	40–65	4.0–8.0
Activated sludge + extended aeration	0.12–0.25	3.5–5.5	20–35	1200–2000	40–105	35–50	4.0–8.0
Conventional activated sludge + tertiary filtration	0.15–0.30	2.5–4.5	18–26	1200–3100	40–100	50–75	6.0–10.0
Low-rate trickling filter	0.15–0.3	0	0	360–1100	35–80	50–60	4.0–6.0
High-rate trickling filter	0.12–0.25	0	0	500–1900	35–80	50–60	4.0–6.0
Rotating biological contactor	0.1–0.2	0	0	330–1500	20–75	50–60	4.0–6.0

UASB, Upflow anaerobic sludge blanket
Source: Adapted from von Sperling & Chernicharo (2005).

9.1.2 Costs and benefits

One difficulty of traditional economic analysis for wastewater use is, however, that the setting of the system boundaries often leads to many important costs or benefits being overlooked. An example of the magnitude of such costs can be seen by considering centralized wastewater treatment works that discharge treated effluent to a surface water body. In addition to the investment, reinvestment and operation and maintenance costs of the sewer network and treatment plant, other costs should be included. It may be necessary to consider important cost transfer implications where wastewater treatment is concerned. For example, wealthier households may benefit from sewerage, but if the sewage is not treated, this may shift costs on to the poor in terms of adverse health impacts and to society in general in terms of environmental impacts. Frequently, the costs of sewage treatment have not been accounted for during planning. Important "downstream" costs of sewage discharges include drinking-water treatment, degradation of the coastal environment, damage to fishing industries, recreational water pollution and lost tourism revenues. Each one of these external costs may in turn incur further costs.

For systems using wastewater, these additional costs may include the necessary transformation costs to adapt the existing infrastructure, additional hygiene promotion activities, monitoring costs and the need for continued research and development of the system. There is, however, also a large number of direct additional benefits when wastewater is safely used, including:

- the value of the water resource;
- the value of the nutrient resource (see Box 9.1);
- increased household food security;
- better household nutrition;
- income generation (see Box 9.2);
- reduced treatment costs (e.g. it is unnecessary to add expensive processes to wastewater treatment facilities to remove nutrients);
- preserving high-quality water sources for high-priority uses such as drinking-water supply (through the use of wastewater for irrigation water instead of high-quality groundwater or surface water and by not discharging effluents to water sources);
- an improvement of soil structure and fertility;
- reduced energy consumption (in the treatment works as well as for fertilizer production).

In order to account for all these costs and benefits, the boundaries used when evaluating wastewater use systems need to be much broader than they are at present.

Some additional economic considerations include the following:

- Sewerage systems are expensive to build, operate and maintain; less expensive alternatives, such as settled sewage, condominial sewers and other technologies, may be available (see Box 9.3).
- The cost of pumping sewage can be substantial; wastewater treatment facilities should be planned in the same areas where the wastewater can be cost-effectively used with minimal pumping (e.g. ponds could be located downhill of treatment facilities).

Box 9.1 Water and nutrient benefits of wastewater use in irrigation

As an example, a city with a population of 500 000 and water consumption of 200 l/day per person would produce approximately 85 000 m^3/day (30 Mm^3/year) of wastewater, assuming 85% inflow to the public sewerage system. If treated wastewater effluent is used in carefully controlled irrigation at an application rate of 5000 m^3/ha per year, an area of some 6000 ha could be irrigated. Products grown on this land could be sold to help offset the costs of treatment and would provide work opportunities for local residents.

In addition to the economic benefit of the water, the fertilizer value of the effluent is of importance. With typical concentrations of nutrients in treated wastewater effluent from conventional sewage treatment processes as follows:

Nitrogen, 50 mg/l
Phosphorus, 10 mg/l
Potassium, 30 mg/l

and assuming an application rate of 5000 m^3/ha per year, the fertilizer contribution of the effluent would be:

Nitrogen, 250 kg/ha per year
Phosphorus, 50 kg/ha per year
Potassium, 150 kg/ha per year

Thus, all of the nitrogen and much of the phosphorus and potassium normally required for agricultural crop production would be supplied by the effluent. In addition, other valuable micronutrients and the organic matter contained in the effluent will provide benefits.

Source: Pescod (1992).

Box 9.2 Wastewater use in Hyderabad and Secunderabad: food security and livelihoods

Wastewater from the cities of Hyderabad and Secunderabad in India flows into the Musi River. During the dry season, 100% of the flow of the river is sewage from the cities. Wastewater from the cities is used to irrigate an estimated 40 600 ha of cropland. The wastewater is available year-round and allows the cultivation of up to three crops per year. Often it is the only source of water due to population growth and overpumping of the aquifers. Over 95% of the irrigated land is used to grow para grass, which is used to feed water buffalo. One hectare of para grass brings in more money than any other crop (e.g. an average of 2812 euros per hectare per year compared with 833 euros per hectare for leafy vegetables). It is estimated that 40 000 people depend directly or indirectly on the cultivation of para grass for their livelihoods.

All of the farmers who grow vegetables on their irrigated plots retain a part of their produce for their own consumption, and the rest is sold. Many of the leafy vegetable producers engage in barter, where they exchange part of their produce for other vegetables to add variety to their diet. In the urban areas, among vegetable producers, 20% of household income is saved because they do not need to purchase vegetables and because they barter their produce for other vegetables. Most of the households in the urban and periurban area with livestock use wastewater-irrigated para grass as fodder and earn income through the sale of the milk. Typically, 25% of the milk produced (assuming that a household of six members owns one buffalo) is retained for household consumption, and 75% is sold. Many of the urban farmers also grow certain fruits, such as lemon, mango, coconut and custard apple, which they retain for household consumption. In the rural areas, it was found that wastewater-irrigated paddies contribute to almost 43% of household food consumption.

Source: Buechler & Devi (2003).

- Low-cost, effective wastewater treatment technologies are available.
- Combinations of different treatment technologies (e.g. primary sedimentation plus polishing ponds) can increase pathogen removal efficiencies at low cost and provide flexibility for upgrading treatment facilities.
- Users of wastewater and excreta are often willing to pay for access to the wastewater and excreta.
- Wastewater and excreta tariffs may help to foster cost recovery.
- Differential prices for treated wastewater and fresh water may provide an incentive for farmers to use wastewater instead of high-quality freshwater sources.
- Wastewater treatment facilities may be able to recover some treatment costs by growing and selling produce at the facility.
- Crop restriction requires costs for agricultural extension workers or inspectors to visit wastewater use areas.
- The initial costs of drip irrigation may be high, but the benefits from the added health protection, need for less wastewater treatment, reduced water use and higher productivity may well outweigh the costs (see Box 9.4).
- As comfortable, affordable gloves and boots become available, farmers are more likely to use them (van der Hoek et al., 2005).
- Posting warning signs may be a low-cost alternative for preventing access to wastewater-irrigated fields.

Box 9.3 Low-cost sewerage

In many Latin American countries, urban households expect to connect to a networked sewerage system. Sewerage is expensive, because it requires extensive underground pipe networks. The pipes have to be a certain diameter to accommodate peak flows. In crowded urban slums or informal settlements, developing conventional sewerage systems can be very difficult, because planning often takes place after the settlement has been established. Narrow streets and crowded conditions also make it difficult to perform the construction activities needed to lay conventional sewerage networks.

In Brazil, an alternative approach was developed more than 20 years ago and is now adopted in many cities and towns. This approach, known as condominial sewerage, uses smaller pipe diameters that are laid on top of the ground, not under it. Smaller-diameter pipes can be effective when the sewage solids are allowed to settle (e.g. in a septic tank) before they are discharged into the sewerage network. Consequently, they are cheaper to build and operate than conventional sewerage systems. The overall costs of conventional sewerage were found to be three times higher than those for condominial or simplified sewerage systems.

Source: Rizo-Pombo (1996).

Wastewater use systems can influence both the individual economic status and the national economy. If wastewater use is managed properly, health risks are significantly reduced. At the individual (household) level, that means money that would have been spent on caring for or curing a sick person can be used to purchase other health-promoting goods or services (e.g. school fees, more nutritious food, etc.). Time gained through reduced illness can be used for education or income-generating activities. At the national level, less monetary and professional resources are dedicated to treating illnesses, and more tax revenues can be collected from increased economic activity.

Box 9.4 Low-cost drip irrigation techniques

Drip irrigation is an effective health protection measure, but the high capital costs often prevent farmers from using this application technique. However, low-cost drip irrigation techniques have been developed in and introduced in a number of different countries, including Cape Verde and India. Drip irrigation systems can use wastewater if it is treated to an adequate level to prevent emitter clogging. In the early 1990s, FAO set up a pilot project in Cape Verde that utilized drip irrigation systems. The new system increased crop production and saved water, allowing for an expansion of irrigated land and cropping intensity. The project was so successful that a number of private farmers adopted the low-cost drip irrigation techniques. Within six years, 22% of all irrigated land in Cape Verde was irrigated with drip systems. As a result, the production of horticultural crops increased from 5700 t in 1991 to 17 000 t in 1999. It is estimated that a plot of 0.2 ha provides farmers with monthly revenues of US$ 1000.

Sources: Postel (2001); FAO (2002).

9.1.3 Multiple objective decision-making processes

The information from economic analysis forms an important input into decision-making processes. It should be used, however, in conjunction with other information so that other factors and externalities may be taken into account. In order to be able to objectively compare different options for wastewater use systems, there is a need for comprehensive, dynamic, integrated, cost–benefit or multicriteria analyses of all types of systems performed over system life cycles or planning periods. This can be achieved using multiple objective decision-making approaches. These involve establishing a range of criteria that consider all key aspects of the system (e.g. health, environmental, sociocultural, economic and technical aspects) and using these to form a basis for decision-making.

A range of different quantification methods can be used in multiple-criteria approaches outside of estimated monetary values, with perhaps DALYs being used to measure health effects and a range of different measurable indicators (e.g. the use of natural resources, discharge to water bodies, etc.) for the environment. Sociocultural aspects, such as the appropriateness of the system or its legal acceptability, can be qualitatively assessed, as can technical issues, such as system robustness or its compatibility with existing systems. The appraisal of a specific project should involve a comparison not only of one system with another, but also of possible variants of the same scheme — for instance, the use of wastewater for different purposes (unrestricted irrigation, restricted irrigation, industrial, non-potable uses).

9.2 Financial feasibility

To ensure sustainable services and cost recovery of wastewater use systems, appropriate financing mechanisms are needed. In drawing up such financing mechanisms, allowances should be made not only for the investment, reinvestment and operation and maintenance of the system, but also for the opportunity and environmental costs and the system's external impacts on individuals and communities (Cardone & Fonseca, 2003).

Resources are needed to ensure institutional capacity building and skills development, monitoring and assessment and the development of an enabling environment for wastewater use. The latter includes awareness-raising campaigns, hygiene promotion, etc. Most of these activities are of a public nature, with both the broader community and the individual households benefiting. Financing for wastewater use, however, mainly comes from two sources: the individual or household and an external source, such as government (Evans, 2004). Trying to mobilize individual household financial resources for activities targeted to the broader community has, however, proven difficult. This raises one of the main challenges of developing financing mechanisms for wastewater use: How can the needs, interests and finances of individuals and households be effectively coordinated and reconciled with those at the community/national level? Ideally, this should be achieved in a way to recover costs, but also to ensure equitable access to resources, particularly for poorer members of society.

Financing mechanisms and institutional responsibilities for collecting user fees or assessing fines are specified in legislation (see chapter 10). Where wastewater is distributed by a separate agency from that which collects and treats it, a charge of some sort is normally payable. Charges are also levied when the wastewater is distributed to individuals.

The level of these charges must be decided at the planning stage. The government must decide whether the charges should be set at a level to cover only the operation and maintenance costs or set higher to recover the capital costs of the scheme as well. While it is, of course, desirable to ensure the maximum recovery of costs, an important consideration is to avoid discouraging the permitted use of wastewater. Some prior investigation of the willingness and ability to pay is therefore essential in determining not only the level of charges, but also the frequency, timing and means of payment. For instance, an annual charge payable after the harvest season may be the easiest to collect.

It may be possible to develop an increased demand for the wastewater by effective marketing. However, the results of a marketing campaign should not be anticipated when setting the initial level of charges, which can be increased progressively as demand is developed.

On the other hand, farmers may sometimes be willing to share in the investment in treatment works that are a prerequisite to obtaining use permits. Their contribution may be in cash or in the form of land for treatment and storage facilities. Experiences in Peru have indicated that farmers may sometimes be willing to perform operational and maintenance tasks associated with treatment, storage and conveyance of wastewater as in-kind contributions to the running costs of the scheme (Bartone & Arlosoroff, 1987).

A farmer will pay for wastewater only if its cost is less than that of the cheapest alternative water and the value of the nutrients it contains. How, then, is the cost of the wastewater determined by the agency that sells it? There are three basic approaches to establishing the price of wastewater. It can be related to:

- its production costs (additional treatment and conveyance);
- the benefits derived from its use; or
- some value judgement based on the user's ability or willingness to pay.

If the first option is selected, it should carry the proviso that costs must be no greater than that of the cheapest alternative source of water available to the user. The nutrient value of the wastewater may be included or ignored.

In the case of agriculture, the price for the wastewater is usually based either on the marginal cost of treatment and conveyance or on the value of the nutrient (usually nitrogen) content, whichever is lower. Box 9.5 shows that even poor farmers are often willing to pay for access to wastewater for irrigation. There are several possible ways of charging for the waste, such as per cubic metre, per hour of discharge from a standard sluice or per hectare of irrigated land.

It can also be paid in various ways: as a specific water rate or purchase price, as a renewal fee for an abstraction permit, as a surcharge on the land rent or as a deduction from the price of centrally marketed crops.

Box 9.5 Payment for access to wastewater

In Pakistan, the right to use wastewater for agriculture costs money (Ensink, Simmons & van der Hoek, 2004). In Quetta, farmers paid US$ 12 000 per year for wastewater, a price that is 2.5 times greater than that of fresh water. In many areas of Pakistan, just the possibility of having wastewater available for irrigation (as opposed to fresh water) makes fees increase from US$ 171 to US$ 351–940 per year, since it allows the harvest of three crops per year instead of one and increases the economic benefits to the household by US$ 300 (Ensink, Simmons & van der Hoek, 2004; Ensink et al., 2004).

Financial considerations regarding different types of health protection measures are discussed below.

Wastewater treatment facilities are expensive to build; the capital investment required exceeds the resources of many municipalities, so it is usually met, together with the cost of the sewerage system, by grants or loans from the central government. The operating costs, on the other hand, can usually be met from a municipal tax or water tariff. The costs of treatment are usually justified for environmental pollution control. In some cases, the costs of treatment systems can be offset by the sale of agricultural products from the system.

However, the treatment of wastewater to a standard of quality adequate for use in agriculture may involve additional costs for construction and maintenance. Some of these additional costs can be met by the sale of the treated wastewater from the fee for the permit allowing its use. In practice, however, the prices charged for the wastewater and the fees levied for permits are often determined by what farmers are able and willing to pay (see Box 9.5). In such cases, the difference may be considered as a government subsidy to promote the safe use of wastewater. The cost of conveyance infrastructure (pipes, channels) and pumping costs also need to be considered in the cost of wastewater provision.

The demands of produce restriction for the purpose of health protection sometimes run against the incentives of the market; fresh vegetables may be more valuable than fodder crops. A producer who complies with produce restriction regulations that prohibit certain crops may make less money than one who disobeys them. This should be considered in the initial planning stage and during a market feasibility analysis.

Regulations, however, have to be enforced, which has associated costs. The enforcement is normally carried out by the body that issues permits to use the wastewater or by local staff of the Ministry of Health. In either case, enforcement of produce restrictions is only one of many tasks performed by the staff responsible, so the cost is usually included in the budget that supports their salaries, transport, etc. However, this is not an excuse for neglecting the cost of establishing an efficient enforcement system. Produce restriction may mean that less needs to be spent on treatment, but it will not be effective if adequate financial provision is not made for its enforcement.

Sprinkler irrigation, which potentially causes more widespread contamination with wastewater than other methods, generally requires less preparation of the land than surface irrigation. If surface or subsurface irrigation is chosen to minimize contamination, the land can often be prepared more easily and cheaply by a central organization than by individual farmers. Alternatively, farmers can be assisted with the loan or hire of the necessary equipment. Since preparation of the fields helps the farmers avoid other expenditure, the cost can be recovered from them in the same way as other irrigation costs — through land rent, water charges or permit fees. Since localized irrigation uses less water and can produce higher yields, farmers themselves may find it worthwhile to change to this method if there are obvious benefits (see Box 9.4). Low-cost drip irrigation systems have been developed and used in Cape Verde and India (see Box 9.4; Postel, 2001; FAO, 2002).

9.3 Market feasibility

In planning for wastewater use, it is important that the market feasibility be assessed. Market feasibility may refer to the ability to sell (treated) wastewater to producers, or it can refer to the marketability of products grown with wastewater (see Table 9.2). For selling treated wastewater, it is important to have an idea of how much people are willing and able to pay. Assessing the market feasibility is particularly important when produce restriction in agriculture is being considered as a partial health protection measure. Producers should be consulted as to which products can be restricted. If farmers or market gardeners cannot make a suitable return on the products that they are allowed to raise, then produce or waste application restrictions are likely to fail.

Table 9.2 Market feasibility: planning questions

Product for sale	Key questions
Treated wastewater	• What is the price for the treated wastewater that people are willing and able to pay?
	• What is the demand in the project area for treated wastewater?
	• Are there extra costs required to get the treated wastewater to where it will be used (e.g. pumping costs, transport, etc.)?
Produce	• Are products acceptable to consumers?
	• Can producers earn acceptable returns with restricted application and produce?
	• Is the project capable of supplying products that meet market quality criteria (e.g. microbial standards for products to be exported)?

Any product derived from the treated wastewater must also be acceptable to the consumers. If the public perception of these products is negative, even if the quality meets WHO or national quality criteria, then producers still may not be able to sell their products. If agricultural products will require post-harvesting processing, the cost and availability of these services need to be considered. In some cases, it will be necessary to market products to increase demand and profit potential.

10
POLICY ASPECTS

The safe management of wastewater use in agriculture is facilitated by appropriate policies, legislation, institutional frameworks and regulations at the international, national and local levels. In many countries where wastewater use in agriculture takes place, these frameworks are lacking. This chapter looks at different country-level strategies for developing appropriate frameworks at each level that will help to encourage the safe use of wastewater in agriculture. It is important that countries create appropriate policies based upon the specific conditions that occur nationally.

As Figure 10.1 shows, policy is the overall framework that sets national development priorities. It can be influenced by international policy decisions (e.g. MDGs, Commission on Sustainable Development), international treaties or commitments (e.g. the United Nations Environment Programme's Global Programme of Action for the Protection of the Marine Environment from Land-based Activities) or multilateral development institutions. Policy leads to the creation of relevant legislation. Legislation establishes the responsibilities and rights of different stakeholders — that is, the institutional framework. The institutional framework determines which agency has the lead responsibility for creating regulations (often as part of a consultative process among ministries) and who has the authority to implement and enforce the regulations.

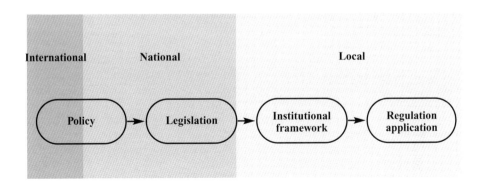

Figure 10.1
Policy framework

10.1 Policy

According to Elledge (2003), policy is the set of procedures, rules and allocation mechanisms that provide the basis for programmes and services. Policies set priorities, and strategies allocate resources for their implementation. Policies are implemented through four types of policy instruments:

1) *Laws and regulations:* Laws generally provide the overall framework. Regulations provide the more detailed guidance. Regulations are rules or governmental orders designed to control or govern behaviour and often have

the force of law. Regulations for wastewater use can cover a wide range of topics, including the practices of service providers, design standards, tariffs, treatment requirements, water quality requirements, monitoring requirements, crop restrictions, environmental protection and contracts. These regulations, especially treatment and water quality standards, have to be adapted to local conditions.

2) *Economic measures:* Examples of economic measures are user charges, subsidies, incentives and fines. User charges, or tariffs, are charges that households and enterprises pay in exchange for the removal of wastewater. Subsidies are allocations in cash or kind to communities and households for establishing recommended types of sanitation facilities or services. Fines are monetary charges imposed on enterprises and people for unsafe disposal, emissions and/or risky hygienic behaviours and practices, which are a danger to people and the environment.

3) *Information and education programmes:* These programmes include public awareness campaigns and educational programmes designed to generate demand and public support for efforts to expand sanitation and hygiene services.

4) *Assignment of rights and responsibilities for providing services:* National governments are responsible for determining the roles of national agencies and the appropriate roles of the public, private and non-profit sectors in programme development, implementation and service delivery.

10.1.1 International policy

International policy may affect the creation of national wastewater use policies. Countries agree to treaties, conventions, International Development Targets, etc. that may commit them to carry out certain actions. For example, countries may have commitments with respect to the MDGs (as described in chapter 1) or the Commission on Sustainable Development or in relation to reducing the use and/or contamination of water resources that cross international boundaries (e.g. by requiring less freshwater abstraction or by requiring wastewater discharges to be treated to higher qualities to reduce basin-wide contamination).

Another major issue is the worldwide export of food. As described in chapter 4, the WTO recognizes the rights of countries to establish standards for the safety of foods imported into their countries. Food products raised in compliance with the WHO *Guidelines for the safe use of wastewater, excreta and greywater* are internationally recognized as being developed within an appropriate risk management framework. This can help to facilitate international trade in food products produced with wastewater and excreta.

10.1.2 National wastewater use policies

Policy priorities for each country are necessarily different to reflect local conditions. National policy on the use of wastewater in agriculture needs to consider various issues, including:

- the health implications of wastewater use in agriculture (requirement for a health impact assessment prior to large-scale project implementation; see Annex 3) and setting of appropriate standards and regulations;
- water scarcity;
- wastewater availability now and in the future;

- locations where wastewater is generated;
- the acceptability of wastewater use in agriculture;
- the extent and types of wastewater use currently practised;
- the ability to effectively manage wastewater use safely;
- downstream impacts if wastewater is not used for agriculture;
- number of people dependent upon wastewater use in agriculture for their livelihoods;
- trade implications of exporting crops produced with wastewater.

10.1.3 Wastewater in integrated water resources management

In many arid and semi-arid countries, the renewable freshwater resources available are already heavily exploited. Countries with less than 1700 m^3 of fresh water per person are considered to be water-stressed, while countries with less than 1000 m^3 of fresh water per person face water scarcity (Hinrichsen, Robey & Upadhyay, 1998).

Wastewater is increasingly being viewed in the greater context of integrated water resources management, especially in arid and semi-arid areas. Wastewater is often a reliable water resource, with constant flows even in the dry season. The use of wastewater in agriculture should figure more prominently in water resources management, because it enables communities to reserve higher-quality water resources (e.g. groundwater or uncontaminated surface water) for uses such as drinking-water supply. The use of wastewater as a supplementary water resource is important in many communities in arid or semi-arid regions (see Box 10.1).

Box 10.1 Wastewater as an input into integrated water resource management — Case study: Israel

Oron (1998) estimates that Israel has 1.8–2.0 km^3 of renewable freshwater resources available per year — i.e. less than 300 m^3 per person (Arlosoroff, 2002). Israel is affected by acute and chronic water scarcity.

The Israel Water Commission (2002) estimated that the total freshwater withdrawal for Israel was 1.9 km^3 in 2000, accounting for 95–106% of all renewable freshwater resources. In a drought year, virtually all of the renewable freshwater resources may be withdrawn.

With freshwater resources stretched to the limit, it is necessary to preserve the best-quality water for uses such as drinking-water supply. The best-quality fresh water comes from several aquifers (Nativ & Issar, 1988). Some of these sources are threatened by saline intrusion and contamination from surface activities — e.g. nitrate leaching from agriculture (Oron, 1998).

In Israel, 79% of fresh water is used for agriculture, while domestic use (16%) and industrial use (5%) account for the rest (Gleick, 2000). In the future, less fresh water will be available for agriculture as the population becomes larger and more affluent and water use increases (Oron, 1998). New freshwater sources will have to be identified and developed. Israel is planning to add to freshwater supplies by desalinating seawater and saline groundwater.

In 1999, 337 × 10^6 m^3 of wastewater was treated (Israel Ministry of the Environment, 2002). In the same year, 80% of the treated wastewater (270 × 10^6 m^3) was used in agriculture (Fedler, 1999). The volume of treated effluents used in agriculture (270 × 10^6 m^3) is nearly equal to the volume of Israel's second largest freshwater aquifer — the Coastal Aquifer — at 283 × 10^6 m^3 (Nativ & Issar, 1988) and thus represents a substantial water resource for the country.

Israel has increased its available freshwater resources by 14% by using wastewater in agriculture. Arlosoroff (2002) predicts that 100% of the total wastewater flow will be used in agriculture by 2010.

Box 10.1 (continued)

Israel manages its wastewater within the broader context of all available water resources. All freshwater resources are closely monitored, and over the years concerted efforts to maximize water use efficiency have reduced the use of water per capita. Water conservation techniques have been applied in agriculture, in urban areas and in industry. The economic value of agricultural production per unit of water has increased fivefold since 1950 (Arlosoroff, 2002). This is largely due to the adoption of more water-efficient irrigation technologies such as drip irrigation and by concentrating production on high-value crops (Arlosoroff, 2002).

Israel has tried to maximize its flexibility for using wastewater by requiring high levels of treatment and developing trading instruments and a water allocation policy that facilitate the exchange of fresh water for treated effluents for use in irrigation (Arlosoroff, 2002).

In addition to the use of wastewater in agriculture, treated wastewater is often used to recharge aquifers to prevent saline intrusion and restore depleted aquifers. Treated wastewater is often stored above and below the ground in reservoirs until it is needed.

10.2 Legislation

Legislation may both facilitate the safe use of wastewater by, for example, creating economic incentives for wastewater treatment and use facilities and create oversight responsibilities. In many cases, it may be sufficient to amend existing legislation, but sometimes new legislation is required. The following areas deserve attention:

- define institutional responsibilities or allocate new powers to existing bodies;
- establish roles and relationships between national and local governments in the sector;
- create rights of access to and ownership of wastewater, including public regulation of its use (see Box 10.2);
- establish land tenure;
- develop public health and agricultural legislation: wastewater quality standards, produce restrictions, application methods, occupational health, food hygiene, etc.

Box 10.2 Water access rights improve health

Giving people access and rights to water is an important step for improving health at the household and community levels through better nutrition and food supply. Many countries lack legal frameworks that ensure access to water rights, especially for the poor. To improve access to water, FAO (2002) suggests that legal reforms that cover the following issues are needed in many countries:

- allocation of water resources between different users, particularly those in rural and urban areas;
- minimizing conflict between those who use the resource for water supply and those who use it for waste disposal;
- promotion of efficient water use;
- regulation of use of wastewater so that it can be safely used;
- reduction of the role of government in rural water projects, increasing the importance of local user groups and removal of impediments to charging for water and recovering costs;
- evolution of systems of land tenure towards written and individual or group titles;
- ensuring legal access to land and water for female heads of household and women generally;
- creation or improvement of an effective water rights administration to manage the water sector in general and the rural water sector in particular.

Sources: IPTRID (1999); FAO (2002).

10.2.1 Institutional roles and responsibilities

Enabling legislation may be required to establish a national coordinating body for wastewater use and to set up local bodies to manage individual schemes. These will require authority either to charge for the wastewater they distribute or to sell any produce. Working within an existing institutional framework may be preferable to creating new institutions.

At the national level, wastewater use in agriculture is an activity that touches the responsibilities of several ministries or agencies. Examples of ministries or agencies that may have jurisdiction over the use of wastewater in agriculture might include:

- *Ministry of Agriculture:* overall project planning; management of state-owned land; installation and operation of irrigation infrastructure; agricultural research and extension, including training; control of marketing.
- *Ministry of Environment:* sets wastewater treatment and effluent quality standards based on environmental concerns; establishes practices for protecting water resources (both surface waters and groundwaters) and the environment; establishes monitoring and analytical testing protocols.
- *Ministry of Health:* health protection, particularly establishment of quality standards and standards for "good practice" (for treated wastewater; products; health protection measures), monitoring methods and schedules for treated wastewater; monitoring implementation of health protection measures; validation of health protection measures for small-scale wastewater irrigation; health impact assessment of new wastewater projects; health education; disease surveillance and treatment.
- *Ministry of Water Resources:* integration of wastewater use into water resources planning and management.
- *Ministry of Education:* develop school curricula concerning sanitation and personal and domestic hygiene and safe practices related to the use of wastewater in agriculture
- *Ministry of Public Works/Local Government:* excreta and wastewater collection, treatment and use.
- *Ministry of Finance and Economic Planning:* economic and financial appraisal of projects; import control (equipment, fertilizers); development of financing mechanisms for wastewater conveyance and treatment and use infrastructure.

Other ministries and government agencies — for example, those concerned with land tenure, rural development, cooperatives and women's affairs — may also be involved.

Cooperation between the relevant agencies is required, particularly between the technical staff involved. Some countries, especially those in which there is water scarcity, may find it advantageous to establish an executive body, such as an interagency technical standing committee, under the aegis of a leading ministry (Agriculture or Water Resources), or possibly a separate organization (with both government and private funding sources), such as an Office for Wastewater Recycling, to be responsible for programmatic development, planning and management.

In many countries, a simple ad hoc committee may be sufficient. Alternatively, existing organizations, such as a National Water Board, may be given responsibility for wastewater use in agriculture, or parts of it. Such an organization should then convene a committee of representatives from the different agencies having sectoral responsibilities. Setting up an interagency or interministerial committee will help to inform others of the challenges or opportunities facing the introduction or strengthening of wastewater use.

In countries with a regional or federal administration, such arrangements for interagency collaboration will be important at the regional or state level. Whereas the general framework of wastewater use policy and standards may be defined at the national level, the regional body will have to interpret and add to these in the light of local conditions.

The local body managing a scheme, or at least the agency collecting the wastewater, often will be under municipal control. If wastewater use is to be promoted in the context of a national policy, this implies careful coordination and definition of the relationship between local and national governments. On the one hand, it may be necessary for the national government to offer incentives to local authorities to promote safe wastewater use; on the other hand, sanctions of some sort may have to be applied to ensure that schemes are implemented without undue risk to public health.

Local governments should be given the authority to develop their own regulations. For example, they should have the ability to collect fees for wastewater treatment or other services, issue permits, conduct inspections, develop produce restrictions, inspect markets, develop decentralized wastewater treatment and use facilities, etc.

Local authorities should have the ability to issue permits for the use of wastewater in agriculture from a public conveyance network. Permits may be issued by the local agricultural or water resources administration, local governments or the body controlling the wastewater distribution system. In many urban and periurban areas the use of wastewater (frequently untreated) for irrigation is widespread. These activities often arise spontaneously and are usually not controlled by local health authorities. Because of the small scale and dispersion of these operations, it may be difficult to provide proper oversight. Local authorities may be able to establish permitting requirements for land use contingent upon the implementation of specified health protection measures — i.e. the observance of sanitary practices regarding application methods, produce restriction and exposure control.

It is common for the body administering the distribution of wastewater to deal with the landowners through users' associations, which may develop from traditional institutions. Permits to use the wastewater can then be issued to the associations, simplifying the administrative task of dealing separately with a large number of small users. Under such an arrangement, the task is also delegated to the associations of enforcing the regulations that must be complied with for a permit to be renewed.

A joint committee or management board, which may include representatives of these associations as well as any particularly large users, the authorities that collect and distribute the wastewater and also the local health authorities, is required. Even in small-scale organizations, some arrangement, such as a committee with community representatives, is important for the users to participate in the management of the project.

In some cases, farmers will be able to directly negotiate contracts for a specified supply of treated wastewater with the utility that treats the wastewater.

10.2.2 Rights of access

Farmers will be reluctant to install infrastructure or treatment facilities unless they have some confidence that they will continue to have access to the wastewater. This access may be regulated by permits and dependent on efficient or sanitary practice by the farmer. In Mexico, the authorities' power to withhold water from farmers who do not comply with crop restrictions is a major factor in their success. Legislation may therefore be required to define the users' rights of access to the wastewater and the powers of those entitled to allocate or regulate those rights (see Box 10.3).

Box 10.3 Rights to wastewater

Customary rights to water are widely recognized. Thus, the present use of wastewater for agriculture may create rights even if it is not a planned activity and does not fulfil health and environmental norms. These rights can conflict with future planned wastewater use projects, especially if treated wastewater is expected to be sold at a higher price than that paid by the original user of the wastewater. For example, in Mexico, the development of a new wastewater treatment plant caused problems for traditional downstream users of the wastewater. The new treatment plant was able to treat the wastewater to a high quality standard and, as part of its planned cost recovery activities, has been investigating potential sales of the water to industrial users. Untreated wastewater has traditionally been discharged into canals and used for downstream irrigation. Mexico issues water concession titles, which guarantee a landowner access to water. However, only 30% of the wastewater-irrigated land has a concession title linked to it. If the wastewater treatment facility goes through with water sales to industrial users, a significant portion of the water might be diverted from downstream users. Since many of the users do not have officially recognized water rights, they will lose their livelihoods (Silva-Ochoa & Scott, 2004).

In Pakistan, a large number of court cases initiated by local water utilities or sanitation agencies have been brought against local farmers, challenging their rights to use wastewater resources. The outcome of these court cases was that farmers were forced either to pay for wastewater or to abandon its use. In Faisalabad, a group of wastewater farmers successfully appealed against one of these court orders once they proved that they had no access to another suitable water source (Ensink et al., 2004).

10.2.3 Land tenure

Security of access to wastewater is worth little without security of land or water tenure. Existing tenure legislation is likely to be adequate for most eventualities, although it may be necessary to define the ownership of virgin land newly brought under cultivation. If it is decided to amalgamate individual agricultural farms under a single management, powers of compulsory purchase may be needed.

10.2.4 Public health

The area of public health includes rules governing produce restrictions and methods of application, as well as quality standards for treated wastewater used in agriculture, product quality standards and other health protection measures discussed in chapter 5 of these Guidelines. The factors affecting the feasibility of enforcing crop restrictions, discussed in chapter 5, are relevant to both new and existing wastewater use schemes. Consumers also have the right to expect safe food products (see Box 10.4).

Box 10.4 Consumers' rights to safe produce

Consumers have the right to demand safe food. Public health concerns have led to several court cases in Pakistani cities (Ensink et al., 2004). In Quetta, after a trial, the farmers were forced by local residents to test the pathogen content in their products by a national certified laboratory. After demonstrating that their wastewater-irrigated crops were not contaminated, farmers were allowed to continue with the practice. In Hyderabad, farmers and the local municipality have come to an agreement to use wastewater only in crops whose edible parts grow above the ground. Potatoes, onions, carrots and garlic, therefore, cannot be cultivated, although salad crops (e.g. lettuce) are allowed.

New legislation may be needed with regard to the implementation, oversight and monitoring of health protection measures. Public health legislation also covers other aspects of health protection, such as occupational health and food hygiene, water and sanitation services, health promotion, school curriculum development, water resources management and vector control, which may not require new measures but may need to be changed to better reflect specific risks associated with wastewater use in agriculture. Where new wastewater irrigation schemes are proposed or existing activities will be expanded, health impact assessment is often conducted to quantify health impacts on local populations. Health impact assessment is discussed in more detail in Annex 3.

10.3 Regulations

Regulations governing the use of wastewater in agriculture should be practical and focus on protecting public health (other issues will also be relevant, such as environmental protection). Most importantly, regulations should be feasible to implement, given the local circumstances.

A framework of regulations could be set up around the different health protection measures (i.e. wastewater treatment, produce restriction, wastewater application, exposure control, immunization/chemotherapy). Regulations may already exist for some of the protective measures. Without some complementary measures, such as regulations that control market hygiene (e.g. availability of adequate sanitation and safe water supplies, market inspectors, periodic laboratory analysis of wastewater-irrigated crops), safe food products raised in compliance with the wastewater use regulations could easily become recontaminated in the market, mitigating any impact of previous health protection measures that have been implemented (see Table 10.1 for examples of activities that might require regulations).

10.4 Developing a national policy framework

In developing a national policy framework to facilitate safe wastewater use in agriculture, it is important to define the objectives of the policy, assess the current policy environment and develop a national approach.

10.4.1 Defining objectives

The use of wastewater in agriculture can have one or more of several objectives. Defining these objectives is important for developing a national policy framework (Mills & Asano, 1998). The main objectives might be:

- to increase national or local economic development;
- to increase crop production;

Table 10.1 Examples of activities that might be covered in regulations

Activities or components	Regulatory considerations
Wastewater	Access rights, tariffs, management (e.g. municipalities, communities, user groups, etc.)
Conveyance	Agency responsible for building infrastructure and operations and maintenance, pumping costs, delivery trucks
Treatment	Treatment requirements depending upon final use, process requirements
Monitoring	Types of monitoring (e.g. process monitoring, analytical, parameters), frequency, location, financial responsibilities
Wastewater application	Fencing, need for buffer zones, requirements for spray drift control
Produce restrictions	Types of produce permitted, not permitted, enforcement, education of farmers/public
Exposure control	Access control for use areas (e.g. sign posting, fences), protective clothing requirements, provision of water and sanitation facilities for workers, hygiene education responsibilities
Market hygiene	Market inspection, provision of safe water and adequate sanitation facilities at markets
Food safety	Crop analysis for other pathogens and toxic metals, consumer education, beef carcass inspection for *Taenia* cysts

- to augment supplies of fresh water and otherwise take full advantage of the resource value of wastewater;
- to dispose of wastewater in a cost-effective, environmentally friendly manner;
- to improve household income, food security and/or nutrition.

Where wastewater is already used, sub-objectives might be to incorporate health and environmental safeguards into management strategies or improve product yields through better practice.

10.4.2 Assessment of policy environment
The right policies can facilitate the safe use of wastewater in agriculture. Current policies often already exist that affect wastewater use in agriculture, both negatively and positively. Conducting an assessment of current policies is often helpful for developing a new national policy or for revising existing policies. The assessment should take place at two levels: from the perspective of both a policy-maker and a project manager. Policy-makers will want to assess the national policies, legislation, institutional framework and regulations to ensure that they meet the national wastewater use objectives (e.g. maximize economic returns without endangering public health or the environment). Project coordinators will want to ensure that current and future wastewater use schemes will be able to comply with all relevant national and local laws and regulations.

The main considerations are:

- *Policy:* Are there clear policies on the use of wastewater in agriculture? Is wastewater use in agriculture encouraged or discouraged?

- *Legislation:* Is wastewater use governed in legislation? What are the rights and responsibilities of different stakeholders?
- *Institutional framework:* Which ministry/agency, mass organizations, etc. have the authority to control the use of wastewater in agriculture, at the national level and at the district/community level? Are the responsibilities of different ministries/agencies clear? Is there one lead ministry, or are there multiple ministries/agencies with overlapping jurisdictions? Which ministry/agency is responsible for developing regulations? Which ministry/agency monitors compliance with regulations? Which ministry/agency enforces the regulations?
- *Regulations:* Do regulations exist? Are the current regulations adequate to meet wastewater use objectives (protect public health, prevent environmental damage, meet produce quality standards for domestic and international trade, preserve livelihoods, conserve water and nutrients, etc.)? Are the current regulations being implemented? Is regulatory compliance being enforced?

It is easier to make regulations than to enforce them. In drafting new regulations (or in choosing which existing ones to enforce), it is important to plan for the institutions, staff and resources necessary to ensure that the regulations are followed. It is important to ensure that the regulations are realistic and achievable in the context in which they are to be applied. It will often be advantageous to adopt a gradual approach or to test a new set of regulations by persuading a local administration to pass them as by-laws before they are extended to the rest of the country.

10.4.3 Developing national approaches based on the WHO Guidelines

Developing national approaches for safe wastewater use practices based on the WHO Guidelines will protect public health the most when they are integrated into comprehensive public health programmes that include other sanitary measures, such as health and hygiene promotion and improving access to safe drinking-water and adequate sanitation. For example, if the Guidelines are followed during crop production but there is recontamination of the crops at the market, then some of the potential health gains are likely to be erased. Other complementary programmes, such as chemotherapy campaigns, should be accompanied by health promotion/education to change behaviours that lead to intestinal helminth infection and the transmission of other diseases.

National approaches need to be adapted to the local sociocultural, environmental and economic circumstances, but should be aimed at progressive improvement of public health. Interventions that address the greatest local health threats first should be given the highest priority. As resources and new data become available, additional health protection measures can be introduced. Box 10.5 illustrates some steps that might be used to develop a progressive national approach for increasing the safety of waste-fed agriculture.

10.4.4 Research

Research on minimizing health impacts associated with wastewater use in agriculture should be conducted at national institutions, universities or other research centres. It is important to conduct research at the national level, because data concerning local conditions are the most important for developing effective health protection measures and may well vary considerably between countries. Pilot schemes can be developed to

Box 10.5 Developing a national approach to wastewater use in agriculture

Approaches to ensure the safe use of wastewater in agriculture should be based on knowledge of local practices, the health implications of these practices and the need to comply with existing legislation/regulation. The first step is often to assess the situation.

Assess the situation
Examples of the types of information that might be helpful in developing an approach are presented below:

- the availability and types of wastewater treatment available;
- the types of agricultural products grown in the area (e.g. eaten cooked or raw);
- techniques for wastewater conveyance/application in agriculture (e.g. pipes, lined channels, unlined channels, pumping requirements, carts and trucks, proximity to local communities, presence of fences, signs, etc.);
- human exposure to wastewater during agricultural practices (e.g. do workers wear protective clothing? do they practise good hygiene? are hygiene and sanitation facilities available at the field level?);
- hygienic conditions of current harvesting techniques and during storage and transport of produce to markets;
- practices in markets where crops are sold (e.g. is there access to safe water and adequate sanitation facilities in markets? do vendors practise good hygiene? is safe water used to wash/freshen produce?).

Public health risks vary from place to place. It is important to understand what health problems may arise in relation to wastewater use. Schistosomiasis occurs only in limited geographic areas but may be an important disease locally. Also, the incidence of vector-borne diseases will vary and should be considered in relevant situations. Information on local public health priorities can be obtained through scientific studies of disease, review of clinical data, outbreak information and prevalence data and interviews with health staff (doctors, nurses, pharmacists) and farmers. There should also be an effort to quantify positive health impacts — for example, on household nutrition and food security.

Involve stakeholders
When possible, relevant stakeholders should be involved in the development of public health approaches. Without their involvement, health protection measures are less likely to succeed. Stakeholders can be involved in the development of policies through participation in national or district-level workshops or through agricultural extension outreach activities.

Strengthen national/local capacity
The implementation of health protection measures will require both national and local institutional oversight. In some cases, institutional capacities may need to be defined or strengthened. Local health authorities should understand their responsibilities for implementing, monitoring, enforcing and promoting health protection measures.

Phased implementation of health protection measures
Health protection measures can be progressively phased in over time if resources are not available. The first measures to be implemented should try to address the greatest public health priorities first. For example, in areas where intestinal helminth infections are endemic, initial steps might be to encourage farmers to wear shoes, to keep their children out of wastewater-irrigated areas or to grow only crops that are eaten cooked. Development of educational materials and local workshops to educate farmers about how to reduce helminth infections could be initiated quickly. Similar programmes could be implemented at markets to improve food hygiene. Wastewater treatment might be initiated over time with progressive upgrades of the system until it is capable of achieving the WHO microbial pathogen reduction targets discussed in chapter 4.

investigate feasible health protection measures and answer production-related questions. In situations where wastewater irrigation is practised in small-scale diffuse facilities, often at the household level, national research may be used to validate health protection measures and then develop guidelines and standards to be used by small-scale farmers. Research results should be disseminated to various groups of stakeholders in a form that is useful to them.

A pilot project is particularly useful in countries with little or no experience of managing wastewater use in agriculture or when the introduction of new techniques is envisaged. Health protection is an important consideration, but there are other questions that are difficult to answer without local experience of the kind a pilot project can give. These questions are likely to include important technical, social and economic aspects. A pilot scheme can help to identify potential health risks and develop ways to control them.

Pilot projects should be planned — that is, a variety of crops (both old and new) should be investigated, with different application rates of wastewater. Information is required not only on yields but also on microbial contamination levels, uptake of toxic metals in plants, the types and concentrations of toxic chemicals and pathogens typically present in local wastewater and effects on the environment.

A pilot project should operate for at least one growing season, or at least one year if production through the seasons is to be investigated. It should be carefully planned so that the work involved is not underestimated and can be carried out correctly; otherwise, repetition in the following year is required. After the experimental period, a successful pilot project may be translated into a demonstration project with training facilities for local operators and farmers.

11

Planning and implementation of wastewater use programmes require a comprehensive progressive approach that responds to the greatest health priorities first. Strategies for planning should include elements on communication to stakeholders, interaction with stakeholders and the collection and use of data. This chapter describes key considerations for planning and implementation of wastewater use programmes at the national level.

Additionally, planning for projects at a local level requires an assessment of several important underlying factors. The sustainability of wastewater use in agriculture relies on the assessment and understanding of eight important factors. These eight factors — health, economic feasibility, social impact and public perception, financial feasibility, environmental impact, market feasibility, institutional feasibility and technical feasibility — have been described in previous chapters. A brief description of how these factors relate to planning and implementation of wastewater use projects is included in this chapter.

The protection of public health in wastewater irrigation requires the development and use of mechanisms for promoting improvement. This is an important planning aspect. The focus on improvement (whether as an investment priority at the regional or national level, development of hygiene education programmes or enforcement of compliance) will depend on the nature of the wastewater use practices and the types of problems identified (WHO, 2004a). A checklist of mechanisms for improvement of wastewater use in agriculture is given below:

✓ *Establishing national priorities:* When the most common problems and shortcomings in wastewater use have been identified, national strategies can be formulated for improvements and remedial measures; these might include changes in training (of managers, administrators, extension workers or field staff), rolling programmes for improvement or changes in funding strategies to target specific needs.

✓ *Establishing regional priorities:* Regional or local health agencies can determine the communities in which to work and which improvement activities are priorities; public health criteria should be considered when priorities are set.

✓ *Establishing hygiene education programmes:* Many of the health-related issues associated with wastewater use in agriculture are related to personal hygiene and food hygiene and cannot be solved by technology alone. The solutions to many of these problems are likely to require participatory educational and promotional activities.

✓ *Auditing of systems and upgrading:* Wastewater use systems should be audited or inspected. The results of these audits can be used to encourage farmers to improve their practices. Enforcement of local regulations to improve health protection measures may be difficult with small-scale producers. It may be more productive to work with farmers through extension workers to improve practices by educating them about health protection measures and risk reduction strategies.

✓ *Ensuring community operation and maintenance:* Support should be provided by a designated authority to enable community members to be trained so that

they are able to assume responsibility for the operation and maintenance of small-scale and community wastewater use operations.
✓ *Establishing public awareness and information channels:* Publication of information on public health aspects of wastewater use in agriculture can encourage farmers to follow good practices, mobilize public opinion and response and reduce the need for regulatory enforcement, which should be an option of last resort.

In order to make best use of limited resources, it is advisable to start with a basic programme that develops in a planned manner. An example of a step-by-step approach, with actions to be taken at initial, intermediate and advanced phases, is described below:

- **Initial phase**
    — Establish requirements for institutional development.
    — Provide training for staff involved in the programme.
    — Define the role of participants (e.g. agricultural extension staff, local health authorities, food safety inspectors, etc.).
    — Develop health protection measures suitable for the area.
    — Implement health protection measures in priority areas.
    — Monitor performance, but limit verification monitoring to a few essential parameters and known hazards of the greatest importance.
    — Establish reporting, filing and communication systems.
    — Advocate improvements according to identified priorities.
    — Establish reporting to local communities, media and regional authorities.
    — Establish liaison with communities; identify community roles in developing health protection measures and means for promoting community participation.

- **Intermediate phase**
    — Train staff involved in the programme.
    — Establish and expand systematic implementation of health protection measures.
    — Expand access to analytical capability for monitoring (often by means of regional laboratories, national laboratories being largely responsible for analytical quality control and training of regional laboratory staff).
    — Develop capacity for statistical analysis of data.
    — Establish a national database.
    — Identify common problems, and promote activities to address them at regional and national levels.
    — Expand reporting to include interpretation at the national level.
    — Draft or revise health-based targets for wastewater use in agriculture.
    — Use legal enforcement where necessary.
    — Involve communities routinely in the development and implementation of health protection measures.

- **Advanced phase**
    — Institutionalize a staff training programme.
    — Establish routine testing for all health-related parameters at defined frequencies.

— Use a national risk management framework for wastewater use in agriculture.
— Improve wastewater use practices on the basis of national and local priorities, hygiene education and enforcement of standards.
— Establish regional databases compatible with the national database.
— Disseminate data and other information at all levels (local, regional and national).
— Involve communities routinely in the development and implementation of health protection measures.

11.1 Reporting and communication

An important element of a safe wastewater use programme is the sharing of information with stakeholders. It is useful to establish appropriate systems of communication with all relevant stakeholders. Proper communication involves both the provision of information and the solicitation of feedback from interested parties. The ability to improve wastewater use practices is highly dependent on the ability to analyse and present information in a meaningful way to different target audiences (see Box 11.1). The target audiences may include:

- public health officials at local, regional and national levels;
- organizations or utilities that manage the collective treatment of wastewater;
- local administrations;
- communities and agricultural producers; or
- local, regional and national authorities responsible for development planning and investment.

11.2 Interaction with community and consumers

Community participation is a desirable component of the planning and implementation of wastewater use programmes. Communities often share both the benefits of wastewater use and exposure to the hazards. The community represents a resource that can be drawn upon for local knowledge and experience. They are the people who are likely to first notice health problems associated with wastewater use and thus can help to solve the problems. Communication strategies should include provision of summary information to product consumers and producers and establishment and involvement of consumer associations at the local, regional and national levels.

It may not always be feasible to provide information directly to an entire community. Thus, it may be appropriate to use community organizations, where they exist, to provide an effective channel for providing feedback and other information to users. By using local organizations to relay information, it is often easier to initiate a process of discussion and decision-making within the community. The most important elements in working with local organizations are to ensure that the organization selected can access the whole community and can initiate discussion on the health protection measures selected and used in wastewater use programmes.

Box 11.1 Communicating health issues

A key issue in the planning process is the communication of important health issues to different stakeholders. Communicating health-related issues to the public and policy-makers should be based on scientific evidence, transformation of the evidence into meaningful information, the development of feasible solutions, impact assessment and engagement and communication with key stakeholders. These are discussed below.

- *Evidence* of a particular environmental or health problem or issue develops. This may be via formal scientific research or analysis or via the monitoring of various environmental and health indicators. Alternatively, evidence may surface anecdotally, in the media or as a result of a catastrophic event. Usually, the evidence, whether formal or informal, will relate directly to local conditions.

- *Transformation* of formal scientific evidence into evidence that is meaningful to policy-makers and/or the general public takes place. This may be via a process of epidemiological/burden of disease assessment, cost-effectiveness and cost–benefit analysis, risk assessment or the aggregation of environmental and health monitoring data into a few key indicators that are readily understandable to decision-makers.

- *Solutions* (i.e. policy alternatives) are considered, along with a discussion of the environmental and health problems. For politicians, the emphasis on or discussion of problems that have no apparent solution may be politically unappealing. Conversely, problems that have solutions may be transformed into political capital.

- *Impact assessment* must occur, to consider the evidence in light of existing and proposed policies. That process may be formalized as part of a health impact assessment (see Annex 3), a loan process, a poverty reduction strategy, a national plan or a budget debate. Alternatively, it may be a completely informal process. In all cases where government articulates policy explicitly, some sort of "impact assessment" is taking place.

- *Engagement* of key decision-makers and stakeholders takes place, considering new evidence and new policy options. That engagement may be facilitated by the activities of local nongovernmental organizations and academic institutions, the activities of a local or international champion or processes triggered by international and intergovernmental agencies, including new conventions or protocol agreements. Commitment by key decision-makers to consider new evidence may require attitude change on the personal, as well as the institutional, level. This change usually occurs incrementally.

- *Communication* of the health risks, and the potential solutions or policies that may address the problem, takes place alongside the engagement and impact assessment process. Optimally, that communication should involve actors in government, the media and all interest groups and stakeholders. Communication is most effective when it is "hands-on," demonstrates the tangible results of the intervention and is interactive, not frontal or passive — e.g. getting key decision-makers, media and stakeholders involved in observing or participating in the improvement of wastewater use in agriculture, sampling/tracking water quality results or running through an estimate of savings to health. Communication materials should be multilayered — e.g. one-page briefs for top officials, more detailed backgrounders for the professional level, media materials, etc.

Source: Fletcher (2005).

11.3 Use of data and information

Strategies for regional prioritization are typically of a medium-term nature and have information requirements. While the management of information at a national level is aimed at highlighting common or recurrent health issues, the objective at a regional level is to assign a degree of priority to individual interventions. It is therefore important to derive a relative measure of health risk. Feasible health protection measures that address the hazards associated with the highest relative risks can then be developed and implemented.

In many situations, especially where production occurs at very small scales, wastewater use practices may fail to adequately protect public health. In such circumstances, it is important that realistic goals for progressive improvement are agreed upon and implemented.

11.4 Project planning criteria

Eight criteria should be considered when planning wastewater use projects: health, economic feasibility, social impact and public perception, financial feasibility, environmental impact, market feasibility, institutional feasibility and technical feasibility (see Figure 11.1) (Mills & Asano, 1998). Failure to meet any one of these criteria may cause a project to fail. Meeting all the criteria can help to ensure that the project is sustainable.

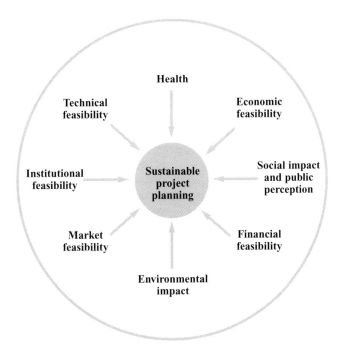

Figure 11.1
Project planning: Eight criteria that impact project success

Most of the eight criteria have been discussed in previous chapters, but a brief discussion of each follows:

1) *Health:* Health is the focus of these Guidelines. Because health issues may vary from one location to the next in the same country, it is important to understand and determine which health issues associated with wastewater use in agriculture are likely to be the most important. Studies are often necessary to identify the key issues. Conducting a health impact assessment prior to the development of new projects or as part of an assessment of ongoing projects is an important planning tool (see Annex 3). Health impact assessment helps to identify populations (e.g. local communities in close proximity to wastewater use areas) that might be at increased risk from different exposures (e.g. vector-borne diseases or schistosomiasis) but may not be considered in other studies. Health impacts, both positive and negative, on the most susceptible populations (e.g. subsistence-level practitioners) need to be considered in the project planning.

2) *Economic feasibility:* Economic feasibility is discussed in chapter 9. Health protection measures that provide the greatest health benefit at the lowest cost should be considered first during project planning.

3) *Social impact and public perception:* These issues were discussed in chapter 7. Cultural practices with respect to wastewater and excreta use, food consumption patterns and other behaviours are very important in the development of health protection measures. It may be very difficult to change long-held beliefs or practices. Health protection measures should be planned to accommodate or even incorporate traditional beliefs and practices. Public perception can be a powerful tool for the acceptance or rejection of a scheme for wastewater use in agriculture. It is important to involve the public in project planning and communicate with different stakeholders. If there is a perceived need for the activity (e.g. because of economic reasons or other factors such as water scarcity), then the public is more likely to accept it.

4) *Financial feasibility:* This is discussed in more detail in chapter 9. Financial planning looks at how a project can be funded. A sustainable project will need to be able to fund the project at all of its stages (i.e. start-up to completion), including equipment, operations and maintenance activities, staff training, monitoring, etc. In some cases, project planners may want to create user's fees or sell products grown in the wastewater-based agricultural system to offset costs.

5) *Environmental impact:* This is discussed in greater detail in chapter 8. Wastewater use often has positive environmental benefits associated with the recycling of important nutrient resources and offering a form of wastewater treatment. However, it can lead to contamination of surface waters and groundwaters, especially if the aquifers are near the surface. Project management to reduce environmental consequences should also assess whether wastewater use activities could lead to increased habitats for vector or snail breeding.

6) *Market feasibility:* The demand for products produced with wastewater should be assessed before they are produced. For example, if one of the health protection measures chosen to meet the health-based target is crop restriction, there has to be sufficient market demand to ensure that the product can be profitably sold in the market (this does not apply to products for household consumption). This also applies to an agency that treats wastewater and wants to create a user fee to recover costs. Treated wastewater can only be sold at a price that farmers are willing and able to pay.

7) *Institutional feasibility:* Project planners should understand the legal and regulatory requirements concerning wastewater use in agriculture. They should be aware of what national and local institutions control wastewater-based agricultural activities and involve them in the planning process. Institutional feasibility is further discussed in chapter 10.

8) *Technical feasibility:* Wastewater use projects should be technically feasible to succeed. Technologies include aspects such as hardware used in the treatment, storage, distribution and use of wastewater and other aspects, such as technical support services and technical training. The most sustainable technologies will be cost effective, upgradable and easy to operate and maintain with local resources. The main technical aspects that should be considered during planning are listed in Box 11.2.

Box 11.2 Technical information to be included in a project plan

- Current and projected generation rates of the wastewater, proportion of industrial effluents, dilution by surface water
- Existing and required wastewater treatment facilities, pathogen removal efficiencies, physicochemical quality
- Existing and required land areas: size, location, soil types, proximity to nearby villages
- Evaporation, especially in waste stabilization ponds (impacts salinity and need for dilution water)
- Conveyance of treated wastewater to farms
- Storage requirements for the wastewater
- Wastewater application rates and methods
- Types of crops to be grown, and their requirements for wastewater quality
- Estimated yields of crops per hectare of land per year
- Strategies for health protection

11.4.1 Support services

Various support services to farmers are particularly relevant to the implementation of health protection measures, and detailed consideration should be given to them at the planning stage. They include the following:

- machinery (sales and servicing, or hire);
- pumps, fences, protective clothing, etc.;
- facilities for processing crops;
- extension and training;
- marketing services, especially where new products are to be introduced or new land is to be brought into productive use;
- primary health care, possibly including regular health checks for workers and their families.

11.4.2 Training

Training requirements must be carefully evaluated at the planning stage, and it may often be necessary to start training programmes, especially for farmers and treatment facility operators, before the project begins, in order to ensure that adequately trained staff is available. Sewage treatment plant operators require on-the-job training in all aspects of the operation of the treatment plant, delivery systems and pumping stations; farmers will need training in agricultural methods most suitable for wastewater use; and technicians will require training in sample collection and analysis.

Similarly, the likely need for agricultural extension services must be estimated and provision made for them to be available to farmers after implementation of the project. Extension officers will themselves need training in the methods appropriate to health protection, as will the staff responsible for enforcing sanitary regulations regarding crop restriction, occupational health, food hygiene, etc.

REFERENCES

AATSE (2004). *Water recycling in Australia*. Melbourne, Australian Academy of Technological Sciences and Engineering.

Ackers ML et al. (1998). An outbreak of *Escherichia coli* O157:H7 infections associated with leaf lettuce consumption. *Journal of Infectious Diseases*, 177:1588–1593.

ACTG (1999). *ACT wastewater reuse for irrigation. Environment protection policy*. Canberra, Australian Capital Territory Government (BDM 99/0415; http://www.environment.act.gov.au/Files/wastewaterreuseforirrigationeppword.doc).

Ait Melloul A, Hassani L (1999). *Salmonella* infection in children from the wastewater-spreading zone of Marrakesh city (Morocco). *Journal of Applied Microbiology*, 87:536–539.

Albonico M et al. (1995). Rate of reinfection with intestinal nematodes after treatment of children with mebendazole or albendazole in a highly endemic area. *Transactions of the Royal Society for Tropical Medicine and Hygiene*, 89:538–541.

Al Khateeb N (2001). Sociocultural acceptability of wastewater reuse in Palestine. In: Faruqui NI, Biswas AK, Bino MJ, eds. *Water management in Islam*. Ottawa, International Development Research Centre/United Nations University Press.

Allen RG et al. (1998). *Crop evapotranspiration — guidelines for computing crop water requirements*. Rome, Food and Agriculture Organization of the United Nations (FAO Irrigation and Drainage Paper 56).

Alloway BJ, Morgan H (1986). The behaviour and availability of cadmium, nickel, and lead in polluted soils. In: Assink JW, van den Brink, eds. *Contaminated soil*. Dordrecht, Martinus Nifhoff Publishers, pp. 101–113.

Anderson J et al. (2001). Climbing the ladder: a step by step approach to international guidelines for water recycling. *Water Science and Technology*, 43(10):1–8.

Arlosoroff S (2002). *Integrated approach for efficient water use — Case study: Israel*. Paper presented at the World Food Prize International Symposium "From the Middle East to the Middle West: Managing Freshwater Shortages and Regional Water Security," Des Moines, IA, 24–25 October 2002 (http://www.worldfoodprize.org/Symposium/02Symposium/2002presentations/Arlosoroff.pdf).

Armon R et al. (1994). Residual contamination of crops irrigated with effluent of different qualities: a field study. *Water Science and Technology*, 30(9):239–248.

Armon R et al. (2002). Surface and subsurface irrigation with effluents of different qualities and presence of *Cryptosporidium* oocysts in soil and on crops. *Water Science and Technology*, 46(3):115–122.

Arthur JP (1983). *Notes on the design and operation of waste stabilization ponds in warm climates of developing countries*. Washington, DC, World Bank (Technical Paper No. 7).

Asano T, ed. (1998). *Wastewater reclamation and reuse*. Lancaster, PA, Technomic Publishing Company.

Asano T, Levine AD (1998). Wastewater reclamation, recycling, and reuse: an introduction. In: Asano T, ed. *Wastewater reclamation and reuse*. Lancaster, PA, Technomic Publishing Company, pp. 1–56.

Asano T et al. (1992). Evaluation of the California wastewater reclamation criteria using enteric virus monitoring data. *Water Science and Technology*, 26(7–8):1513–1524.

Ayers RS, Westcot DW (1985). *Water quality for agriculture.* Rome, Food and Agriculture Organization of the United Nations (FAO Irrigation and Drainage Paper 29, Revision 1; http://www.fao.org/docrep/003/T0234E/T0234E00.htm).

Ayres RM et al. (1992a). Contamination of lettuces with nematode eggs by spray irrigation with treated and untreated wastewater. *Water Science and Technology*, 26(7–8):1615–1623.

Ayres RM et al. (1992b). A design equation for human intestinal nematode egg removal in waste stabilization ponds. *Water Research*, 26:863–865.

Barnes KK et al. (2002). *Water-quality data for pharmaceuticals, hormones, and other organic wastewater contaminants in U.S. streams, 1999–2000.* Iowa City, IA, United States Geological Survey (USGS Open File Report 02-94; http://toxics.usgs.gov/pubs/OFR-02-92/).

Bartone CR, Arlosoroff S (1987). Reuse of pond effluents in developing countries. *Water Science and Technology*, 19(12):289–297.

Bartram J, Fewtrell L, Stenström T-A (2001). Harmonised assessment of risk and risk management for water-related infectious disease: an overview. In: Fewtrell L, Bartram J, eds. *Water quality: Guidelines, standards and health — Assessment of risk and risk management for water-related infectious disease.* London, IWA Publishing on behalf of the World Health Organization.

Bastos RKX, Mara DD (1995). The bacteriological quality of salad crops drip and furrow irrigated with waste stabilization pond effluent: an evaluation of the WHO guidelines. *Water Science and Technology*, 31(12):425–430.

Baumhogger W (1949). Ascariasis in Darmstadt and Hessen as seen by a wastewater engineer. *Zeitschrift für Hygiene und Infektions Krankheiten*, 129:488–506.

Beaglehole R, Bonita R, Kjellström T (1993). *Basic epidemiology.* Geneva, World Health Organization.

Belmont MA et al. (2004). Treatment of domestic wastewater in a pilot-scale natural treatment system in central Mexico. *Ecological Engineering*, 23:299–311.

Benham-Blair & Affiliates, Inc., Engineering Enterprises, Inc. (1979). *Long-term effects of land application of domestic wastewater: Dickinson, North Dakota, slow rate irrigation site.* Washington, DC, United States Environmental Protection Agency (EPA-600/2-79-144).

Beuchat LR (1998). *Surface decontamination of fruits and vegetables eaten raw: a review.* Geneva, World Health Organization (Report No. WHO/FSF/FOS/98.2).

BGS-CNA (1998). *Impact of wastewater reuse on groundwater in the Mezquital Valley, Hidalgo State, Mexico. Final report.* Mexico City, British Geological Survey and National Water Commission (CNA).

Blumenthal U, Peasey A (2002). *Critical review of epidemiological evidence of the health effects of wastewater and excreta use in agriculture.* Unpublished document prepared for the World Health Organization by London School of Hygiene and Tropical Medicine, London (available upon request from WHO, Geneva).

Blumenthal U et al. (2000a). Guidelines for the microbiological quality of treated wastewater used in agriculture: recommendations for revising WHO guidelines. *Bulletin of the World Health Organization*, 78(9):1104–1116.

Blumenthal UJ et al. (2000b). *Guidelines for wastewater reuse in agriculture and aquaculture: recommended revisions based on new research evidence.* London, Water and Environmental Health at London and Loughborough; and London, London School of Hygiene and Tropical Medicine (WELL Study Task No. 68, Part 1).

Blumenthal UJ et al. (2001). The risk of enteric infections associated with wastewater reuse: the effect of season and degree of storage of wastewater. *Transactions of the Royal Society of Tropical Medicine and Hygiene*, 95:1–7.

Blumenthal UJ et al. (2003). *Risk of enteric infections through consumption of vegetables with contaminated river water*. London, London School of Hygiene and Tropical Medicine.

Bole J, Bell R (1978). Land application of municipal sewage wastewater: yield and chemical composition of forage crops. *Journal of Environmental Quality*, 7:222–226.

Bouhoum K, Schwartzbrod J (1998). Epidemiology study of intestinal helminthiasis in a Marrakech raw sewage spreading zone. *Zentralblatt für Hygiene und Umweltmedizin*, 200:553–561.

Bouwer H (1991). Groundwater recharge with sewage effluent. *Water Science and Technology*, 23:2099–2108.

Bouwer H, Chaney RL (1974). Land treatment of wastewater. In: Brady NC, ed. *Advances in agronomy. Vol. 26.* New York, Academic Press, pp. 133–176.

Brackett RE (1987). Antimicrobial effect of chlorine on *Listeria monocytogenes*. *Journal of Food Protection*, 50:999–1003.

Bridgeman J (2004). Public perception towards water recycling in California. *The Journal*, 18(3):150–154.

Buechler S, Devi G (2003). *Household food security and wastewater-dependent livelihood activities along the Musi River in Andhra Pradesh, India*. Unpublished document prepared for the World Health Organization by the International Water Management Institute, Colombo (available upon request from WHO, Geneva).

Cabaret J et al. (2002). The use of urban sewage sludge on pastures: the cysticercosis threat. *Veterinary Research*, 33:575–597.

California State Water Resources Control Board (2003). *Recycled water use in California*. Sacramento, CA, California State Water Resources Control Board, Office of Water Recycling
(http://www.swrcb.ca.gov/recycling/docs/wrreclaim1_attb.pdf).

Calvo M et al. (2004). [Prevalence of *Cyclospora* sp., *Cryptosporidium* sp., microsporidia and fecal coliform determination in fresh fruit and vegetables consumed in Costa Rica.] *Archivos Latinoamericanos de Nutricion*, 54(4):428–432 (in Spanish).

Camann DE, Moore BE (1987). Viral infections based on clinical sampling at a spray irrigation site. In: *Implementing water reuse. Proceedings of water reuse symposium IV*. Denver, CO, American Water Works Association, pp. 847–863.

Camann DE et al. (1986a). *Lubbock land treatment system research and demonstration project. Vol. IV. Lubbock Infection Surveillance Study*. Research Triangle Park, NC, United States Environmental Protection Agency (EPA Publication No. EPA/600/2-86/027d).

Camann DE et al. (1986b). *Infections and spray irrigation with municipal wastewater: the Lubbock Infection Surveillance Study*. Research Triangle Park, NC, United States Environmental Protection Agency (unpublished document).

Capra A, Scicolone B (2004). Emitter and filter tests for wastewater reuse by drip irrigation. *Agricultural Water Management*, 68:135–149.

Cardone R, Fonseca C (2003). *Thematic overview paper: Financing and cost recovery*. Delft, IRC International Water and Sanitation Centre (http://www.irc.nl/page/113).

Carr R, Bartram J (2004). The Stockholm framework for guidelines for microbial contaminants in drinking water. In: Cotruvo J et al., eds. *Waterborne zoonoses: Identification, causes, and control*. London, IWA Publishing on behalf of the World Health Organization.

Carr R, Blumenthal U, Mara D (2004). Health guidelines for the use of wastewater in agriculture: developing realistic guidelines. In: Scott C, Faruqui NI, Raschid-Sally L, eds. *Wastewater use in irrigated agriculture: confronting the livelihood and environmental realities*. Wallingford, CAB International in association with the International Water Management Institute and International Development Research Centre, pp. 41–58.

Chang AC, Page AL, Asano T (1995). *Developing human health–related chemical guidelines for reclaimed wastewater and sewage sludge applications in agriculture*. Geneva, World Health Organization.

Chang AC et al. (2002). *Developing human health–related chemical guidelines for reclaimed water and sewage sludge applications in agriculture*. Geneva, World Health Organization (unpublished document).

Chen Z-S (1992). Metal contamination of flooded soils, rice plants, and surface waters in Asia. In: Adriano DC, ed. *Biogeochemistry of trace metals*. Boca Raton, FL, Lewis Publishers, pp. 85–108.

Chen ZS, Lee GJ, Liu JC (1997). Chemical remediation treatments for soils contaminated with cadmium and lead. In: Iskandar IK et al., eds. *Proceedings of the fourth international conference on the biogeochemistry of trace elements, Berkeley, CA*. Berkeley, CA, University of California, pp. 421–422.

Chorus I, Bartram J, eds. (1999). *Toxic cyanobacteria in water: a guide to their public health consequences, monitoring and management*. London, E & FN Spon on behalf of the World Health Organization, Geneva.

Cifuentes E (1998). The epidemiology of enteric infections in agricultural communities exposed to wastewater irrigation: perspectives for risk control. *International Journal of Environmental Health Research*, 8:203–213.

Cifuentes E et al. (2000a). Health risk in agricultural villages practicing wastewater irrigation in Central Mexico: perspectives for protection. In: Chorus I et al., eds. *Water sanitation & health*. London, IWA Publishing, pp. 249–256.

Cifuentes E et al. (2000b). The risk of *Giardia intestinalis* infection in agricultural villages practicing wastewater irrigation in Mexico. *American Journal of Tropical Medicine and Hygiene*, 62(3):388–392.

Clancy JL et al. (1998). UV light inactivation of *Cryptosporidium* oocysts. *Journal of the American Water Works Association*, 90(9):92–102.

Cordy G et al. (2003). Persistence of pharmaceuticals, pathogens, and other organic wastewater contaminants when wastewater is used for ground-water recharge. In: *Proceedings of the third international conference on pharmaceuticals and endocrine disrupting chemicals in water, Minneapolis, MN, 19–21 March*. Westerville, OH, National Ground Water Association.

Cornish GA, Lawrence P (2001). *Informal irrigation in peri-urban areas: a summary of findings and recommendations*. Wallingford, United Kingdom Department for International Development (Report OD 144 HR).

Cox S (2000). *Mechanisms and strategies for phytoremediation of cadmium*. Fort Collins, CO, Colorado State University, Department of Horticulture. (http://lamar.colostate.edu/~samcox/BIBLIOGRAPHY.html, accessed 16 January 2003).

Crook J et al. (1992). *Guidelines for water reuse*. Cambridge, MA, Camp Dresser & McKee, Inc.

Cross P (1985). *Health aspects of nightsoil and sludge use in agriculture and aquaculture. Part I: Existing practices and beliefs in the utilization of human excreta.* Duebendorf, International Reference Centre for Waste Disposal (Report No. 04/85).

Curtis TP, Mara DD, Silva SA (1992). Influence of pH, oxygen & humic substances on ability of sunlight to damage fecal coliforms in waste stabilization pond water. *Applied and Environmental Microbiology*, 58(4):1335–1345.

Darrell V (2002). *Rule Development Committee issue research report draft, organic loading rates.* Tumwater, WA, Washington State Department of Health, Wastewater Management Program (http://www.doh.wa.gov/ehp/ts/WW/TechIssueReports/T-3aOrganicLoading-VSD.doc).

Day A, Tucker T (1977). Effects of treated wastewater on growth, fiber, protein and amino acid content of sorghum grains. *Journal of Environmental Quality*, 6(3):325–327.

Day A, Taher F, Katterman F (1975). Influence of treated municipal wastewater on growth, fibre, acid soluble nucleotide, protein and amino acid content in wheat grain. *Journal of Environmental Quality*, 4(2):167–169.

Degens B et al. (2000). Irrigation of an allophanic soil dairy factory effluent for 22 years: responses of nutrient storage and soil biota. *Australian Journal of Soil Research*, 38:25–35.

Downs T et al. (2000). Effectiveness of natural treatment in a wastewater irrigation district of the Mexico City region: a synoptic field survey. *Water Environment Research*, 72(1):4–21.

Drakatos P et al. (2002). Antagonistic action of Fe and Mn in Mediterranean-type plants irrigated with wastewater effluents following biological treatment. *International Journal of Environmental Studies*, 59(1):125–132.

Drewes JE, Heberer T, Reddersen K (2002). Fate of pharmaceuticals during indirect potable reuse. *Water Science and Technology*, 46(3):73–80.

Duqqah M (2002). *Treated sewage water use in irrigated agriculture: theoretical design of farming systems in Seil Al Zarqa and the Middle Jordan Valley in Jordan* [PhD thesis]. Wageningen, Wageningen University.

EcoSanRes (2005). *Closing the loop on phosphorus.* Stockholm, Stockholm Environment Institute, Ecological Sanitation Research Programme (EcoSanRes Fact Sheet 4).

Edwards P (1992). *Reuse of human wastes in aquaculture: a technical review.* Washington, DC, United Nations Development Programme, World Bank Water and Sanitation Program.

El-Gohary F et al. (1993). Assessment of the performance of oxidation pond system for wastewater reuse. *Water Science and Technology*, 27(9):115–123.

Elledge MF (2003). *Thematic overview paper: sanitation policies.* Delft, IRC International Water and Sanitation Centre (http://www.irc.nl/page/3273).

Engineering Science (1987). *Final report: Monterey wastewater reclamation study for agriculture.* Berkeley, CA, Engineering Science.

Ensink J, Simmons J, van der Hoek W (2004). Wastewater use in Pakistan: the cases of Haroonabad and Faisalabad. In: Scott CA, Faruqui NI, Raschid-Sally L, eds. *Wastewater use in irrigated agriculture: confronting the livelihood and environmental realities.* Wallingford, CAB International in association with the International Water Management Institute and International Development Research Centre, pp. 91–102.

Ensink J et al. (2004). A nationwide assessment of wastewater use in Pakistan: an obscure activity or a vitally important one? *Water Policy*, 6:197–206.

Ensink J et al. (2005). High risk of hookworm infection among wastewater farmers in Pakistan. *Transactions of the Royal Society of Tropical Medicine and Hygiene*, 99:809–818.

EUREPGAP (2004). *Guideline: MRL, crop protection and water quality information sources*. Cologne, EUREPGAP (Code reference MRL 1.3GL).

Evans B (2004). *Whatever happened to sanitation? — Practical steps to achieving a core development goal*. Prepared for Norwegian Ministry of the Environment (http://www.dep.no/md/engelsk/csd12/topics/022021-990432).

FAO (2002). *Crops and drops: making the best use of water for agriculture*. Rome, Food and Agriculture Organization of the United Nations.

Farid M et al. (1993). The impact of reuse of domestic wastewater from irrigation on groundwater quality. *Water Science and Technology*, 27(9):147–157.

Farooq S, Ansari ZI (1983). Water reuse in Muslim countries — an Islamic perspective. *Environmental Management*, 7(2):119–123.

Faruqui NI, Biswas AK, Bino MJ, eds. (2001). *Water management in Islam*. Ottawa, International Development Research Centre/United Nations University Press.

Faruqi N, Niang S, Redwood M (2004). Untreated wastewater reuse in market gardens: a case study of Dakar, Senegal. In: Scott CA, Faruqui NI, Raschid-Sally L, eds. *Wastewater use in irrigated agriculture: confronting the livelihood and environmental realities*. Wallingford, CAB International in association with the International Water Management Institute and International Development Research Centre, pp. 113–125.

Fattal B, Yekutiel P, Shuval HI (1986). Cholera outbreak in Jerusalem 1970, revisited: the evidence for transmission by wastewater irrigated vegetables. In: Goldsmith JR, ed. *Environmental epidemiology: epidemiological investigation of community environmental health problems*. Boca Raton, FL, CRC Press, pp. 49–59.

Fattal B, Lampert Y, Shuval H (2004). A fresh look at microbial guidelines for wastewater irrigation in agriculture: a risk-assessment and cost-effectiveness approach. In: Scott CA, Faruqui NI, Raschid-Sally L, eds. *Wastewater use in irrigated agriculture*. Wallingford, CAB International in association with the International Water Management Institute and International Development Research Centre, pp. 59–68.

Fattal B et al. (1985). Wastewater reuse and exposure to *Legionella* organisms. *Water Resources*, 19(6):693–696.

Fattal B et al. (1986). Health risks associated with wastewater irrigation: an epidemiological study. *American Journal of Public Health*, 76(8):977–979.

Fattal B et al. (1987). Viral antibodies in agricultural populations exposed to aerosols from wastewater irrigation during a viral disease outbreak. *American Journal of Epidemiology*, 125(1):899–906.

Feachem RG et al. (1983). *Sanitation and disease: health aspects of excreta and wastewater management*. Chichester, John Wiley & Sons (World Bank Studies in Water Supply and Sanitation 3).

Fedler J (1999). *Focus on Israel: Israel's agriculture in the 21st century*. Jerusalem, Israel Ministry of Foreign Affairs

(http://www.mfa.gov.il/mfa/go.asp?MFAH00170, accessed 26 February 2003).

Fewtrell L, Bartram J, eds. (2001). *Water quality: Guidelines, standards and health — Assessment of risk and risk management for water-related infectious disease*. London, IWA Publishing on behalf of the World Health Organization.

Fletcher E (2005). *Environment and health decision-making in a developing country context.* Geneva, World Health Organization/United Nations Environment Programme.

Foster S et al. (2004). *Urban wastewater as groundwater recharge — evaluating and managing the risks and benefits.* Washington, DC, World Bank (Briefing Note 12; http://lnweb18.worldbank.org/ESSD/ardext.nsf/18ByDocName/BriefingNoteNo1 2UrbanwastewaterasGroundwaterRecharge-- evaluatingandmanagingtherisksandbenefits283KB/$FILE/BriefingNote_12.pdf).

Friedel J et al. (2000). Effects of long-term wastewater irrigation on soil organic matter, soil microbial biomass and activities in Central Mexico. *Biology and Fertility of Soils*, 31:414–421.

Frost JA et al. (1995). An outbreak of *Shigella sonnei* infection associated with consumption of iceberg lettuce. *Emerging Infectious Diseases*, 1:26–29.

Future Harvest (2001). *Wastewater irrigation: economic necessity or threat to health and environment?* Consultative Group on International Agricultural Research (http://www.futureharvest.org/earth/wastewater.shtml, accessed 16 October 2001).

Gambrill MP (1990). *Physicochemical treatment of tropical wastewater* [PhD thesis]. Leeds, University of Leeds, School of Civil Engineering.

Geldreich EE, Bordner RH (1971). Fecal contamination of fruits and vegetables during cultivation for processing and marketing: a review. *Journal of Milk and Food Technology*, 34:184–195.

Girovich MJ, ed. (1996). *Biosolids treatment and management: processes for beneficial use.* New York, Marcel Dekker, Inc. (Environmental Science and Pollution Control 18).

Gittinger JP (1982). *Economic analysis of agricultural projects.* Baltimore, MD, Johns Hopkins University Press.

Gleick PH (2000). *The world's water 2000–2001: the biennial report on freshwater resources.* Washington, DC, Island Press.

Grant SB et al. (1996). Prevalence of enterohemorrhagic *Escherichia coli* in raw and treated municipal sewage. *Applied and Environmental Microbiology*, 62(9):3466–3469.

Grimason AM et al. (1993). Occurrence and removal of *Cryptosporidium* spp oocysts and *Giardia* spp cysts in Kenyan waste stabilization ponds. *Water Science and Technology*, 27(3–4):97–104.

Haas CN (1983). Estimation of risk due to low doses of microorganisms: a comparison of alternative methodologies. *American Journal of Epidemiology*, 118(4): 573–582.

Haas CN, Rose JB, Gerba CP (1999). *Quantitative microbial risk assessment.* New York, John Wiley & Sons.

Haas CN et al. (1993). Risk assessment of virus in drinking water. *Risk Analysis*, 13(5):545–552.

Habbari K et al. (2000). Geohelminth infections associated with raw wastewater reuse for agricultural purposes in Beni-Mallal, Morocco. *Parasitology International*, 48:249–254.

Harleman D, Murcott S (2001). An innovative approach to urban wastewater treatment in the developing world. In: *Water21*, June issue. London, IWA Publishing, pp. 44–48.

Havelaar AH, Melse JM (2003). *Quantifying public health risk in the WHO guidelines for drinking-water quality: a burden of disease approach.* Bilthoven, National Institute for Public Health and the Environment (RIVM).

Heberer T, Reddersen K, Mechlinski A (2002). From municipal sewage to drinking water: fate and removal of pharmaceutical residues in the aquatic environment in urban areas. *Water Science and Technology*, 46(3):81–88.

Helmer R, Hespanhol I, eds. (1997). *Water pollution control — a guide to the use of water quality management principles.* London, E & FN Spon on behalf of the United Nations Environment Programme, Water Supply and Sanitation Collaborative Council and the World Health Organization.

Hernandez F et al. (1997). Rotavirus and hepatitis A virus in market lettuce (*Lactuca sativa*) in Costa Rica. *International Journal of Food Microbiology*, 37:221–223.

Hinrichsen D, Robey B, Upadhyay UD (1998). *Solutions for a water-short world.* Baltimore, MD, Johns Hopkins University, School of Public Health (Population Reports, Series M, No. 14).

Hopkins RJ et al. (1993). Seroprevalence of *Helicobacter pylori* in Chile: vegetables may serve as one route of transmission. *Journal of Infectious Diseases*, 168:222–226.

Hurst CJ, Benton WH, Stetler RE (1989). Detecting viruses in water. *Journal of the American Water Works Association*, 8(9):71–80.

Intermediate Technology Consultants (2003). *Low cost micro-irrigation technologies for the poor.* Rugby, Intermediate Technology Consultants.

International Development Enterprises (2005). *Drip irrigation.* Lakewood, CO, IDE-International (http://www.ideorg.org/Page.asp?NavID=211).

IPCS (2002). *Global assessment of the state-of-the-science of endocrine disruptors.* Geneva, World Health Organization, International Programme on Chemical Safety.

IPTRID (1999). *Poverty reduction and irrigated agriculture.* Rome, Food and Agriculture Organization of the United Nations, International Programme for Technology and Research in Irrigation and Drainage (Issues Paper No. 1).

Israel Ministry of the Environment (2002). *Sewage and effluents: amount of raw sewage from treatment plants.* Jerusalem, Israel Ministry of the Environment (http://www.cbs.gov.il/shnaton53/st27_10.pdf, accessed 26 February 2003).

Israel Water Commission (2002). *Water production and consumption, by source and purpose.* Tel Aviv, Israel Water Commission (http://www.cbs.gov.il/shnaton53/st21_06.pdf, accessed 26 February 2003).

IWA Specialist Group (2000). *Constructed wetlands for pollution control: processes, performance, design and operation.* London, IWA Publishing (Scientific and Technical Report No. 8).

Jenkins MB et al. (2002). *Cryptosporidium parvum* oocyst inactivation in three soil types at various temperatures and water potentials. *Soil Biology and Biochemistry*, 34(8):1101–1109.

Jiménez B (2003). Health risk in aquifer recharge with recycled water. In: Aertgeerts R, Angelakis A, eds. *State of the art report: health risks in aquifer recharge using reclaimed water.* Copenhagen, World Health Organization Regional Office for Europe, pp. 54–190 (Report No. EUR/03/5041122).

Jiménez B (2004). El Mezquital, Mexico: The biggest irrigation district that uses wastewater. In: Lazarova V, Bahri A, eds. *Water reuse for irrigation: agriculture, landscapes, and turf grass.* Boca Raton, FL, CRC Press, 456 pp.

Jiménez B (2005). Treatment technology and standards for agricultural wastewater reuse: a case study in Mexico. *Journal of Irrigation and Drainage*, 54:1–11.

Jiménez B, Chávez A (1997). Treatment of Mexico City wastewater for irrigation purposes. *Environmental Technology*, 18:721–730.

Jiménez B, Chávez A (1998). Removal of helminth eggs in an advanced primary treatment with sludge blanket. *Environmental Technology*, 19:1061–1071.

Jiménez B, Chávez A (2002). Low cost technology for reliable use of Mexico City's wastewater for agricultural irrigation. *Environmental Technology*, 9(1–2):95–108.

Jimenez B, Chávez A (2004). Quality assessment of an aquifer recharged with wastewater for its potential use as drinking source: "El Mezquital Valley" case. *Water Science and Technology*, 50(2):269–273.

Jiménez B et al. (2001). The removal of a diversity of micro-organisms in different stages of wastewater treatment. *Water Science and Technology*, 43(10):155–162.

Jiménez B, Siebe C, Cifuentes E (2004). [Intentional and non-intentional reuse of wastewater in the Tula Valley.] In: Jimenez B, Marin L, eds. [*The water in Mexico: a view from the Academy.*] Mexico City, Mexican Academy of Sciences, pp. 35–55 (in Spanish).

Juanicó M, Dor I (1999). *Hypertrophic reservoirs for wastewater storage and reuse: ecology, performance, and engineering design.* Heidelberg, Springer Verlag.

Juanicó M, Milstein A (2004). Semi-intensive treatment plants for wastewater reuse in irrigation. *Water Science and Technology*, 50(2):55–60.

Kapperud G et al. (1995). Outbreak of *Shigella sonnei* infection traced to imported iceberg lettuce. *Journal of Clinical Microbiology*, 33(3):609–614.

Karimi AA, Vickers JC, Harasick RF (1999). Microfiltration goes to Hollywood: the Los Angeles experience. *Journal of the American Water Works Association*, 91(6):90–103.

Katzenelson E, Buiu I, Shuval HI (1976). Risk of communicable disease infection associated with wastewater irrigation in agricultural settlements. *Science*, 194:944–946.

Kay M (2001). *Smallholder irrigation technology: prospects for sub-Saharan Africa.* Rome, Food and Agriculture Organization of the United Nations, International Programme for Technology and Research in Irrigation and Drainage.

Khalil M (1931). The pail closet as an efficient means of controlling human helminth infections as observed in Tura prison, Egypt, with a discussion on the source of *Ascaris* infection. *Annals of Tropical Medicine and Parasitology*, 25:35–62.

Khouri N, Kalbermatten J, Bartone CR (1994). *Reuse of wastewater in agriculture: a guide for planners.* Washington, DC, United Nations Development Programme/World Bank Water and Sanitation Program (Water and Sanitation Report No. 6).

Knobeloch L et al. (2000). Blue babies and nitrate-contaminated well water. *Environmental Health Perspectives*, 108(7):675–678.

Kosek M, Bern C, Guerrant RL (2003). The global burden of diarrhoeal disease, as estimated from studies published between 1992 and 2000. *Bulletin of the World Health Organization*, 81(3):197–204.

Krey W (1949). The Darmstadt ascariasis epidemic and its control. *Zeitschrift für Hygiene und Infektions Krankheiten*, 129:507–518.

Krishnamoorthi KP, Abdulappa MK, Anwikar AK (1973). Intestinal parasitic infections associated with sewage farm workers with special reference to helminths and protozoa. In: *Proceedings of symposium on environmental pollution.* Nagpur, Central Public Health Engineering Research Institute, pp. 347–355.

Landa H, Capella A, Jiménez B (1997). Particle size distribution in an effluent from an advanced primary treatment and its removal during filtration. *Water Science and Technology*, 36(4):159–165.

Lang MM, Harris LJ, Beuchat LR (2004). Survival and recovery of *Escherichia coli* O157:H7, *Salmonella*, and *Listeria monocytogenes* on lettuce and parsley as affected by method of inoculation, time between inoculation and analysis, and treatment with chlorinated water. *Journal of Food Protection*, 67:1092–1103.

Lazarova V et al. (2000). Wastewater disinfection by UV: evaluation of the MS2 phages as a biodosimeter for plant design. In: *Proceedings of the WateReuse Association symposium 2000, Napa, CA, 12–15 September*. Alexandria, VA, WateReuse Association (CD-ROM).

Leach L, Enfield C, Harlin C (1980). *Summary of long-term rapid infiltration system studies*. Washington, DC, United States Environmental Protection Agency (EPA-600/2-80-165).

Lee S et al. (2004). Sorption behaviors of heavy metals in SAT (soil aquifer treatment) system. *Water Science and Technology*, 50(2):263–268.

Ling B (2000). Health impairments arising from drinking water polluted with domestic sewage and excreta in China. In: Chorus I et al., eds. *Water sanitation & health*. London, IWA Publishing, pp. 43–46.

Linnemann CC et al. (1984). Risk of infection associated with a wastewater spray irrigation system used for farming. *Journal of Occupational Medicine*, 26(1):41–44.

Lipton M (1983). *Poverty, under-nutrition and hunger*. Washington, DC, World Bank (World Bank Staff Working Paper No. 597).

Ludwig HF et al. (2005). *Textbook of appropriate sewerage technologies for developing countries*. New Delhi, South Asian Publishers Pvt. Ltd.

Mansell J, Drewes J, Rauch T (2004). Removal mechanisms of endocrine disrupting compounds (steroids) during soil aquifer treatment. *Water Science and Technology*, 50(2):229–237.

Mara DD (2004). *Domestic wastewater treatment in developing countries*. London, Earthscan Publications.

Mara DD, Silva SA (1986). Removal of intestinal nematode eggs in tropical waste stabilization ponds. *Journal of Tropical Medicine and Hygiene*, 89(2):71–74.

Mara DD et al. (1997). *Wastewater storage and treatment reservoirs in northeast Brazil*. Leeds, University of Leeds, School of Civil Engineering, Tropical Public Health Engineering (TPHE Research Monograph No. 12).

Marais GvR (1966). New factors in the design, operation and performance of waste stabilization ponds. *Bulletin of the World Health Organization*, 34:737–763.

Margalith M, Morag A, Fattal B (1990). Antibodies to polioviruses in an Israeli population and overseas volunteers. *Journal of Medical Virology*, 30:68–72.

Marten GC, Larson WE, Clapp CE (1980). Effects of municipal wastewater effluent on performance and feed quality of maize vs. reed canary grass. *Journal of Environmental Quality*, 9(1):137–141.

Mathers CD et al. (2002). *Global burden of disease 2000: Version 2 methods and results*. Geneva, World Health Organization.

Matsuno Y et al. (2004). Assessment of the use of wastewater for irrigation: a case in Punjab, Pakistan. In: Steenvoorden J, Endreny T, eds. *Wastewater re-use and groundwater quality*. Wallingford, International Association of Hydrological Sciences (IAHS Publication 285).

Mead PS et al. (1999). Food-related illness and death in the United States. *Emerging Infectious Diseases*, 5(5):607–625.

Metcalf & Eddy, Inc. (1991). *Wastewater engineering: treatment, disposal and reuse*, 3rd ed. New York, McGraw-Hill.

Metcalf & Eddy, Inc. (2003). *Wastewater engineering: treatment, disposal and reuse*, 4th ed. New York, McGraw-Hill.

Mikkelsen R, Camberato J (1995). Potassium, sulfur, lime and micronutrient fertilizers. In: Rechcigl J, ed. *Soil amendments and environmental quality*. Chelsea, MI, Lewis Publishers.

Mills RA, Asano T (1998). Planning and analysis of wastewater reuse projects. In: Asano T, ed. *Wastewater reclamation and reuse*. Lancaster, PA, Technomic Publishing Company.

Mills WR et al. (1998). Groundwater recharge at the Orange County water district. In: Asano T, ed. *Wastewater reclamation and reuse*. Lancaster, PA: Technomic Publishing Company, pp. 1105–1142.

Monreal J (1993). *Estudio de caso de Chile: evolución de la morbilidad entérica en Chile, luego de la aplicación de medidas de restricción de cultivas en zonas regadas con aguas servidas.* Paper presented at the World Health Organization / Food and Agriculture Organization / United Nations Environment Programme / United Nations Center for Human Settlements Workshop on Health, Agriculture and Environmental Aspects of Wastewater Use, Juitepec, Mexico, 8–12 November 1993.

Montresor A et al. (2002). *Helminth control in school-age children: a guide for managers of control programmes*. Geneva, World Health Organization, 64 pp.

Montresor A et al. (2005). *How to add deworming to vitamin A distribution*. Geneva, World Health Organization (Report No. WHO/CDS/CPE/PVC/2004.11).

Moore BE et al. (1988). Microbial characterization of municipal wastewater at a spray irrigation site: the Lubbock Infection Surveillance Study. *Journal of the Water Pollution Control Federation*, 60:1222–1230.

Morrissey S, Harleman D (1992). Retrofitting conventional primary treatment plants for chemically enhanced primary treatment in the USA. In: Klute R, Hahn H, eds. *Chemical water and wastewater treatment. II. Proceedings of the 5th Gothenburg symposium*. Berlin, Springer-Verlag, pp. 401–416.

Moulton-Hancock C et al. (2000). *Giardia* and *Cryptosporidium* occurrence in groundwater. *Journal of the American Water Works Association*, 92(9):117–123.

Müller EE, Grabow WIK, Ehlers MM (2003). Immunomagnetic separation of *Escherichia coli* O157:H7 from environmental and wastewater in South Africa. *Water SA*, 29(4):427–432.

Murray CJL, Acharya AK (1997). Understanding DALYs. *Journal of Health Economics*, 16:703–730.

Murray CJL, Lopez AD, eds. (1996). *The global burden of disease. Vol. 1*. Cambridge, MA, Harvard School of Public Health on behalf of the World Health Organization and the World Bank.

Najafi P, Mousavi S, Feizi M (2003). Effects of using treated municipal wastewater in irrigation of tomato. *Journal of Agricultural Science and Technology*, 15(1):65–67.

NAS, NAE (1972). *Water quality criteria.* Washington, DC, National Academy of Sciences and National Academy of Engineering, Commission on Water Quality Criteria.

National Research Council (1996). *Use of reclaimed water and sludge in food crop production*. Washington, DC, National Academy Press, pp. 64–65.

National Research Council (1998). *Issues in potable reuse: the viability of augmenting drinking water supplies with reclaimed water*. Washington, DC, National Academy Press.

Nativ R, Issar A (1988). Problems of an over-developed water-system — the Israeli case. *Water Quality Bulletin*, 13(4):126–131, 146.

NRMMC, EPHCA (2005). *National guidelines for water recycling: managing health and environmental risks*. Canberra, Natural Resource Management Ministerial

Council and Environment Protection and Heritage Council of Australia.

Ongley ED (1996). *Control of water pollution from agriculture.* Rome, Food and Agriculture Organization of the United Nations (FAO Irrigation and Drainage Paper 55).

Oragui JI et al. (1987). Removal of excreted bacteria and viruses in deep waste stabilization ponds in northeast Brazil. *Water Science and Technology,* 19:569–573.

Oron G (1998). Water resources management and wastewater reuse for agriculture in Israel. In: Asano T, ed. *Wastewater reclamation and reuse.* Lancaster, PA, Technomic Publishing Company, pp. 757–778.

Oron G et al. (1991). Subsurface microirrigation with effluent. *Journal of Irrigation and Drainage Engineering,* 117(1):25–36.

Oron G et al. (1992). Effect of effluent quality and application method on agricultural productivity and environmental control. *Water Science and Technology,* 26(7–8):1593–1601.

Ortega YR et al. (1997). Isolation of *Cryptosporidium parvum* and *Cyclospora cayetanensis* from vegetables collected from markets of an endemic region in Peru. *American Journal of Tropical Medicine and Hygiene,* 57:683–686.

Pahren H et al. (1979). Health risks associated with land application of municipal sludge. *Journal of the Water Pollution Control Federation,* 51(11):2588–2601.

Parameswaran M (1999). Urban wastewater use. *Plant Biomass Production, Resources, Conservation and Recycling,* 27(1–2):39–56.

Peasey A (2000). *Human exposure to* Ascaris *infection through wastewater reuse in irrigation and its public health significance* [PhD thesis]. London, University of London.

Peasey A et al. (2000). *A review of policy and standards for wastewater reuse in agriculture: a Latin American perspective.* London, Water and Environmental Health at London and Loughborough (WELL Study No. 68, Part II; http://www.lboro.ac.uk/well/).

Pescod M (1992). *Wastewater treatment and use in agriculture.* Rome, Food and Agriculture Organization of the United Nations (FAO Irrigation and Drainage Paper 47).

Peters R, Lee C, Bates D (1980). *Field investigations of overland flow treatment of municipal lagoon effluent.* Vicksburg, MS, United States Army Corps of Engineers, Waterways Experiment Station.

Petterson SA, Ashbolt NJ (2003). *WHO guidelines for the safe use of wastewater and excreta in agriculture: microbial risk assessment section.* Geneva, World Health Organization (unpublished document, available upon request from WHO, Geneva).

Petterson SR, Teunis PFM, Ashbolt NJ (2001a). Modeling virus inactivation on salad crops using microbial count data. *Risk Analysis,* 21:1097–1107.

Petterson SR, Ashbolt NJ, Sharma A (2001b). Microbial risks from wastewater irrigation of salad crops: a screening-level risk assessment. *Water Environment Research,* 72(6):667–672; Errata: *Water Environment Research,* 74(4):411.

Pettygrove GS, Asano T (1985). *Irrigation with reclaimed municipal wastewater — a guidance manual.* Chelsea, MI, Lewis Publishers.

Phene CJ, Ruskin R (1989). *Nitrate management of wastewater with subsurface drip irrigation.* Corte Madera, CA, Geoflow Inc. (http://www.Geoflow.com).

Polak P, Nanes B, Adhikari D (1997). A low cost drip irrigation system for small farmers in developing countries. *Journal of the American Water Resources Association,* 33(1):119–124.

Porter B et al. (1984). An outbreak of shigellosis in an ultra-orthodox Jewish community. *Social Science and Medicine*, 18(12):1061–1062.

Postel S (2001). Growing more food with less water. *Scientific American*, February 2001:34–37.

Prüss A, Havelaar A (2001). The global burden of disease study and applications in water, sanitation, and hygiene. In: Fewtrell L, Bartram J, eds. *Water quality: Guidelines, standards and health — Assessment of risk and risk management for water-related infectious disease*. London, IWA Publishing on behalf of the World Health Organization.

Raschid-Sally L, van der Hoek W, Ranawaka M, eds. (2001). *Wastewater reuse in agriculture in Vietnam: water management, environment and human health aspects*. Proceedings of a workshop held in Hanoi, Viet Nam. Battaramulla, International Water Management Institute (Working Paper 30).

Rashed M et al. (1995). Monitoring of groundwater in Gabal el Asfar wastewater irrigated area (Greater Cairo). *Water Science and Technology*, 32(11):163–169.

Reed S, Thomas R, Kowal N (1980). Long term land treatment, are there health or environmental risks? In: *Proceedings of the ASCE national convention, Portland, OR*. Reston, VA, American Society of Civil Engineers.

Rivera F et al. (1995). Removal of pathogens from wastewater by the root zone method (RZM). *Water Science and Technology*, 32(3):211–218.

Rizo-Pombo JH (1996). The Colombian ASAS system. In: Mara DD, ed. *Low-cost sewerage*. Chichester, John Wiley & Sons.

Robertson LJ, Campbell AT, Smith HV (1992). Survival of *Cryptosporidium parvum* oocysts under various environmental pressures. *Applied and Environmental Microbiology*, 58(11):3494–3500.

Robinson KG, Robinson CH, Hawkins SA (2005). Assessment of public perception regarding wastewater reuse. *Water Science and Technology*, 5(1):59–65.

Rojas-Valencia N et al. (2004). Ozonation by-products issued from the destruction of micro-organisms present in wastewaters treated for reuse. *Water Science and Technology*, 50(2):187–193.

Rose JB, Gerba CP (1991). Use of risk assessment for development of microbial standards. *Water Science and Technology*, 24(2):29–34.

Rose JB et al. (1996). Removal of pathogenic and indicator micro-organisms by a full-scale water reclamation facility. *Water Resources*, 30(11):2785–2797.

Rose JB et al. (1997). Evaluation of microbiological barriers at the Upper Occoquan Sewage Authority. In: *Water reuse conference proceedings, 25–28 February 1996, San Diego, CA*. Denver, CO, American Water Works Association, pp. 291–305.

Sagik BP, Moor BE, Sorber CA (1978). Infectious disease potential of land application of wastewater. In: *State of knowledge in land treatment of wastewater. Vol. 1. Proceedings of an international symposium*. Hanover, NH, United States Army Corps of Engineers, Cold Regions Research and Engineering Laboratory.

Sala L, Serra M (2004). Towards sustainability in water recycling. *Water Science and Technology*, 50(2):1–8.

Schaefer ML et al. (2004). Biological diversity versus risk for mosquito nuisance and disease transmission in constructed wetlands in southern Sweden. *Medical and Veterinary Entomology*, 18(3):256–261.

Schwartzbrod J et al. (1989). Impact of wastewater treatment on helminth eggs. *Water Science and Technology*, 21(3):295–297.

Scott CA, Zarazua JA, Levine G (2000). *Urban-wastewater reuse for crop production in the water-short Guanajuato River basin, Mexico.* Colombo, International Water Management Institute (Research Report 41).

Seabrook BL (1975). *Land application of wastewater in Australia.* Washington, DC, United States Environmental Protection Agency (EPA-430/9-75-017).

Sehgal R, Mahajan RC (1991). Occupational risks in sewage workers. *The Lancet,* 338:1404–1406.

Shahalam A, Abuzahra B, Jaradat A (1998). Wastewater irrigation effect on soil, crop and environment — a pilot scale study at Irbid, Jordan. *Water, Air, and Soil Pollution,* 106(3–4):425–445.

Sheikh B, Cooper RC, Israel KE (1999). Hygienic evaluation of reclaimed water used to irrigate food crops — a case study. *Water Science and Technology,* 40(4–5):261–267.

Shende GB et al. (1985). Status of wastewater treatment and agricultural reuse with special reference to Indian experience and research and development needs. In: Pescod MB, Arar A, eds. *Treatment and use of sewage effluent for irrigation.* London, Butterworths, pp. 185–209.

Shiklomanov IA (1998). *Assessment of water resources and water availability in the world.* New York, United Nations (Report for the Comprehensive Assessment of the Freshwater Resources of the World).

Shuval HI (1993). Investigation of typhoid fever and cholera transmission by raw wastewater irrigation in Santiago, Chile. *Water Science and Technology,* 27(3–4):167–174.

Shuval HI, Lampert Y, Fattal B (1997). Development of a risk assessment approach for evaluating wastewater reuse standards for agriculture. *Water Science and Technology,* 35(11–12):15–20.

Shuval HI, Yekutiel P, Fattal B (1984). Epidemiological evidence for helminth and cholera transmission by vegetables irrigated with wastewater: Jerusalem — a case study. *Water Science and Technology,* 17:433–442.

Shuval HI et al. (1986). *Wastewater irrigation in developing countries: health effects and technical solutions.* Washington, DC, World Bank (Technical Paper No. 51).

Shuval HI et al. (1989). Transmission of enteric disease associated with wastewater irrigation: a prospective epidemiological study. *American Journal of Public Health,* 79(7):850–852.

Sidle RC, Hook JE, Kardos LT (1976). Heavy metal application and plant uptake in a land disposal system for wastewater. *Journal of Environmental Quality,* 5(1):97–102.

Siebe C (1998). Nutrient inputs to soils and their uptake by alfalfa through long-term irrigation with untreated sewage effluent in Mexico. *Soil Use and Management,* 13:1–5.

Siebe C, Fischer W (1996). Effect of long term irrigation with untreated sewage effluents on soil properties and heavy metals absorption of leptosols and vertisols in Central Mexico. *Pflanzenernahrsm Bodenk,* 159:357–364.

Silva-Ochoa P, Scott CA (2004). Treatment plant effects on wastewater irrigation benefits: revisiting a case study in the Guanajuato River Basin, Mexico. In: Scott CA, Faruqui NI, Raschid-Sally L, eds. *Wastewater use in irrigated agriculture: confronting the livelihood and environmental realities.* Wallingford, CAB International in association with the International Water Management Institute and International Development Research Centre.

Simmons RW, Pongsakul P (2002). Toward the development of an effective sampling protocol to "rapidly" evaluate the distribution of Cd in contaminated, irrigated rice-based agricultural systems. In: Kheoruenromne I, ed. *Transactions of the 17th world congress of soil science, Bangkok, 14–21 August 2002.* Vienna, International Union of Soil Science.

Sleigh PA, Mara DD (2003). *Monte Carlo program for estimating disease risks in wastewater reuse.* Leeds, University of Leeds, Water & Environmental Engineering Research Group, Tropical Public Health Engineering (http://www.efm.leeds.ac.uk/CIVE/MCarlo).

Smit J, Nasr J (1992). Urban agriculture for sustainable cities: using wastes and idle land and water bodies as resources. *Environment and Urbanization,* 4(2):141–152.

Sobsey M (1989). Inactivation of health-related micro-organisms in water by disinfection processes. *Water Science and Technology,* 21(3):179–195.

Solomon EB, Yaron S, Matthews KR (2002). Transmission of *Escherichia coli* O157:H7 from contaminated manure and irrigation water to lettuce plant tissue and its subsequent internalization. *Applied and Environmental Microbiology,* 68(1):397–400.

Squire L, Van Der Tak HG (1975). *Economic analysis of projects.* Baltimore, MD, Johns Hopkins University Press.

Srivastava VK, Pandey GK (1986). Parasitic infestation in sewage farm workers. *Indian Journal of Parasitology,* 10(2):193–194.

State of California (2001). *California Code of Regulations, Title 22, Division 4, Chapter 3: Water recycling criteria (Sections 60301–60357).* Sacramento, CA, Office of Administrative Law.

Steen I, Agro K (1998). Phosphorus availability in the 21st century: management of a nonrenewable resource. *Journal of Phosphorus and Potassium,* 217 (http://www.nhm.ac.uk/research-curation/departments/mineralogy/research-groups/phosphate-recovery/p&k217/steen.htm).

Stephenson T et al. (2000). *Membrane bioreactors for wastewater treatment.* London, IWA Publishing.

Stine SW et al. (2005). Application of microbial risk assessment to the development of standards for enteric pathogens in water used to irrigate fresh produce. *Journal of Food Protection,* 68(5):913–918.

Stott R et al. (1994). *An experimental evaluation of potential risks to human health from parasitic nematodes in wastewaters treated in waste stabilization ponds and used for crop irrigation.* Leeds, University of Leeds, Department of Civil Engineering, Tropical Public Health Engineering (TPHE Research Monograph No. 6).

Strauss M (1985). Health aspects of nightsoil and sludge use in agriculture and aquaculture — Part II: Survival of excreted pathogens in excreta and faecal sludges. *IRCWD News,* 23:4–9. Duebendorf, Swiss Federal Institute for Environmental Science and Technology (EAWAG) / Department of Water and Sanitation in Developing Countries (SANDEC).

Strauss M (1996). Health (pathogen) considerations regarding the use of human waste in aquaculture. *Environmental Research Forum,* 5–6:83–98.

Strauss M (2000). *Human waste (excreta and wastewater) reuse.* Prepared for the ETC/Swedish International Development Agency Bibliography on Urban Agriculture. Duebendorf, Swiss Federal Institute for Environmental Science and Technology (EAWAG) / Department of Water and Sanitation in Developing Countries (SANDEC) (http://www.sandec.ch/UrbanAgriculture/documents/reuse_health/Human_waste_ use_ETC_SIDA_UA_bibl.pdf).

Sturbaum GD et al. (1998). Detection of *Cyclospora cayetanensis* in wastewater. *Applied and Environmental Microbiology*, 64(4):2284–2286.

Tanaka H et al. (1998). Estimating the safety of wastewater reclamation and reuse using enteric virus monitoring data. *Water Environment Research*, 70(1):39–51.

Tanji KK, Kielen NC (2002). *Agricultural drainage water quality management in arid and semi-arid areas*. Rome, Food and Agriculture Organization of the United Nations (FAO Irrigation and Drainage Paper No. 61).

Taylor HD et al. (1995). Drip irrigation with waste stabilization pond effluents: solving the problem of emitter fouling. *Water Science and Technology*, 31(12):417–424.

TDR (2004). *TDR diseases*. Geneva, World Health Organization, Special Programme for Research and Training in Tropical Diseases (http://www.who.int/tdr/diseases).

Tiessen H, ed. (1995). *Phosphorus in the global environment: transfers, cycles and management*. New York, John Wiley and Sons (SCOPE 54).

Trang DT et al. (in press) Risks for helminth parasite infection among farmers working with wastewater-fed rice culture in Nam Dinh, Vietnam. *Journal of Water and Health*.

UKWIR (2005). *Framework for developing water reuse criteria with reference to drinking-water supplies*. London, United Kingdom Water Industry Research Limited (UKWIR Report Reference No. 05/WR/29/01).

United Nations General Assembly (2000). *United Nations Millennium Declaration. Resolution A/RES/55/2*. New York, United Nations (http://www.un.org/millennium/declaration/ares552e.pdf).

United Nations Population Division (2000). *World population nearing 6 billion, projected close to 9 billion by 2050*. New York, United Nations Population Division, Department of Economic and Social Affairs (http://www.un.org/esa/population/unpop.htm).

United Nations Population Division (2002). *World urbanization prospects: the 2001 revision*. New York, United Nations Population Division, Department of Economic and Social Affairs (http://www.un.org/esa/population/publications/wup2001/WUP2001report.htm).

USEPA (1981). *Land treatment of municipal wastewater*. Washington, DC, United States Environmental Protection Agency (EPA 625/1-81/013).

USEPA (1990). National sewage sludge survey: availability of information and data and anticipated impacts on proposed regulations; Proposed Rule 40 CFR Part 503. *Federal Register*, 55:47210–47283.

USEPA (1992). *Technical support document for land application of sewage sludge*. Prepared for Office of Water, United States Environmental Protection Agency, by Eastern Research Group, Lexington, MA.

USEPA, USAID (1992). *Guidelines for water reuse*. Washington, DC, United States Environmental Protection Agency and United States Agency for International Development (Technical Report No. 81).

van der Hoek W et al. (2005). Skin diseases among people using urban wastewater in Phnom Penh. *Urban Agriculture Magazine*, 14:30–31.

Vaz da Costa Vargas S, Bastos RKX, Mara DD (1996). *Bacteriological aspects of wastewater irrigation*. Leeds, University of Leeds, Department of Civil Engineering, Tropical Public Health Engineering (TPHE Research Monograph No. 8).

Victorian Government Department of Sustainability and Environment (2004). *Framework for mosquito management in Victoria; a bibliography*. Melbourne.

von Sperling M, Chernicharo CAL (2005). *Biological wastewater treatment in warm climate regions*. London, IWA Publishing.

von Sperling M, Fattal B (2001). Implementation of guidelines: some practical aspects. In: Fewtrell L, Bartram J, eds. *Water quality: Guidelines, standards and health — Assessment of risk and risk management for water-related infectious disease*. London, IWA Publishing on behalf of the World Health Organization, pp. 361–376.

von Sperling M, Bastos RKX, Kato MT (2004). *Removal of* E. coli *and helminth eggs in UASB–polishing pond systems*. Paper presented at the 6th International Water Association international conference on waste stabilization ponds, Avignon, 27 September – 1 October.

von Sperling M, et al. (2003). Evaluation and modelling of helminth egg removal in baffled and unbaffled ponds treating anaerobic effluent. *Water Science and Technology*, 48(2):113–120.

von Westarp S, Chieng S, Schreier H (2004). A comparison between low-cost drip irrigation, conventional drip irrigation and hand watering in Nepal. *Agricultural Water Management*, 64:143–160.

Wang G, Zhao R, Doyle MP (1996). Fate of enterohemorrhagic *Escherichia coli* O157:H7 in bovine faeces. *Applied Environmental Microbiology*, 62:2567–2570.

Ward BK, Irving LG (1987). Virus survival on vegetables spray-irrigated with wastewater. *Water Resources*, 21:57–63.

Ward RL et al. (1989). Effect of wastewater spray irrigation on rotavirus infection rates in an exposed population. *Water Research*, 23(12):1503–1509.

Warner W (2000). The influence of religion on wastewater treatment: a consideration for sanitation experts. *Water*, 21:11–13.

Warnes S, Keevil CW (2003). *Survival of* Cryptosporidium parvum *in faecal wastes and salad crops*. Carlow, Teagasc Irish Agriculture and Food Development Authority (http://www.teagasc.ie/publications/2003/conferences/cryptosporidiumparvum).

Weber B, Juanicó M (2004). Salt reduction in municipal sewage allocated for reuse: the outcome of a new policy in Israel. *Water Science and Technology*, 50(2):17–22

WEF (1996). *Wastewater disinfection*. Alexandria, VA, Water Environment Federation (Manual of Practice No. FD-10).

Westcot DW (1997a). *Quality control of wastewater for irrigated crop production*. Rome, Food and Agriculture Organization of the United Nations (Water Report 10).

Westcot DW (1997b). *Drainage water quality*. In: Madramootoo CA, Johnston WR, Williardson LS, eds. *Management of agricultural drainage water quality*. Rome, Food and Agriculture Organization of the United Nations (Water Report 13).

WHO (1973). *Reuse of effluents: Methods of wastewater treatment and health safeguards. Report of a WHO Meeting of Experts*. Geneva, World Health Organization (Technical Report Series No. 517).

WHO (1975). *Health effects relating to direct and indirect re-use of waste water for human consumption. Report of an international working meeting held in Amsterdam, 13–16 January 1975*. Geneva, World Health Organization, 164 pp. (Technical Paper No. 7).

WHO (1988). *Environmental management for vector control*. Geneva, World Health Organization.

WHO (1989). *Health guidelines for the use of wastewater in agriculture and aquaculture*. Geneva, World Health Organization (Technical Report Series No. 776).

WHO (1992). *Cadmium — environmental aspects*. Geneva, World Health Organization, 156 pp. (Environmental Health Criteria 135).

WHO (1999). *Food safety issues associated with products from aquaculture: report of a joint FAO/NACA/WHO study group*. Geneva, World Health Organization (WHO Technical Report Series No. 883).

WHO (2000a). *Bench aids for the diagnosis of intestinal parasites*. Geneva, World Health Organization.

WHO (2000b). *Human health and dams, the World Health Organization's submission to the World Commission on Dams (WCD)*. Geneva, World Health Organization (Document WHO/SDE/WSH/00.01).

WHO (2000c). Hepatitis A vaccines. *Weekly Epidemiological Record*, 75(5):38–44.

WHO (2000d). *Turning the tide of malnutrition: responding to the challenge of the 21st century*. Geneva, World Health Organization (Report No. WHO/NHD/00.7).

WHO (2001a). *Health impact assessment: harmonization, mainstreaming and capacity building; report of a WHO inter-regional meeting and a partnership meeting held at Esami, Arusha, Tanzania, 31 October – 3 November 2000*. Geneva, World Health Organization (WHO/SDE/WSH/01.07).

WHO (2001b). *Depleted uranium: sources, exposure and health effects*. Geneva, World Health Organization (Report No. WHO/SDE/PHE/01.1).

WHO (2002). *Prevention and control of schistosomiasis and soil-transmitted helminthiasis. Report of a WHO Expert Committee*. Geneva, World Health Organization (WHO Technical Report Series 912).

WHO (2003a). *Guidelines for safe recreational water environments. Vol. 1. Coastal and fresh waters*. Geneva, World Health Organization.

WHO (2003b). *The world health report 2003 — Shaping the future*. Geneva, World Health Organization.

WHO (2003c). *Typhoid vaccine. Fact sheet*. Geneva, World Health Organization (http://www.who.int/vaccines/en/typhoid.shtml).

WHO (2004a). *Guidelines for drinking-water quality*, 3rd ed. Geneva, World Health Organization.

WHO (2004b). *The world health report 2004 — Changing history*. Geneva, World Health Organization.

WHO (2005). *Guidelines for safe recreational water environments. Vol. 2. Swimming pools and similar recreational water environments*. Geneva, World Health Organization.

World Food Programme (1995). *World Food Programme mission statement*. Rome, Food and Agriculture Organization of the United Nations.

Yates MV, Gerba CP (1998). Microbial considerations in wastewater reclamation and reuse. In: Asano T, ed. *Wastewater reclamation and reuse*. Lancaster, PA, Technomic Publishing Company, pp. 437–488.

Yuan Y (1993). Etiological study of high stomach cancer incidence among residents in wastewater irrigated areas. *Environmental Protection Science*, 19(1):70–73.

A1.1 Introduction

In addition to mitigating possible health effects associated with the use of wastewater in agriculture, good irrigation practices will need to be followed to ensure a good crop yield and minimize risks to the environment. Irrigation practices with wastewater or with other water sources are similar and depend on the local conditions, including climate, physical and chemical soil properties, drainage conditions and the salt tolerances of the crops to be grown. Good irrigation practices will vary but are based on:

- water quantity;
- water quality;
- soil characteristics (infiltration, drainage);
- crop selection;
- irrigation techniques (see discussion in chapter 5);
- leaching;
- management practices.

This chapter will provide a brief overview of these subjects. For a more thorough discussion of these topics, see Tanji & Kielen (2002), Pescod (1992) and Ayers & Westcot (1985).

A1.2 Water quantity

The amount of water available for irrigation will ultimately determine what types of crops can be grown and what types of irrigation techniques can be used. Most water applied to crops is lost by evapotranspiration from the plant surface. Therefore, the water required by the crops is usually equal to the amount of water lost by evapotranspiration. The evapotranspiration requirement is largely dependent on crops and climatic factors and thus can be estimated based on local meteorological data (Allen et al., 1998). FAO has developed a computer program (CROPWAT) to help farmers determine crop water requirements based on climatic factors (Pescod, 1992). CROPWAT is available at http://www.fao.org/landandwater/aglw/cropwat.stm. The appropriate quantity of water to use will need to be adjusted for the amount of rainfall, leaching requirements, application losses and other factors (Pescod, 1992).

Crops have different sensitivities to water supply. For example, groundnuts (peanuts) and safflower have low sensitivities to water supply, while rice and bananas have high sensitivities to water supply. For more information on the water requirements and sensitivities to water supply for different crops, see Pescod (1992).

A1.3 Water quality

Often, the limits on concentrations of many chemicals in the wastewater will be determined by crop requirements and not by health concerns (see Table A1.1). The nutrients in wastewater (i.e. nitrogen, potassium, phosphorus, zinc, boron and sulfur) should be present in the right concentrations, or they can damage the crops and/or the environment. For example, wastewater often contains high concentrations of nitrogen. Although plants require nitrogen for growth, excessive nitrogen can cause overstimulation of growth, delayed maturity or poor-quality produce. Plants require different amounts of nitrogen based on their growth stage. In the first stages of growth, plants may require high quantities of nitrogen (in the earliest stages of growth, plants require lots of nitrogen, but may be too small to usefully assimilate all that is applied), but in the later flowering and fruiting stages, they may require less. In some cases, nitrogen levels will need to be adjusted by blending water supplies (Ayers & Westcot, 1985). This is also an important consideration to reduce leaching of nitrate into groundwater supplies, which would pose a potential health risk to consumers of the drinking-water (see chapter 3).

Table A1.1 Water quality for irrigation

Parameter		Units	Degree of restriction on use		
			None	Slight to moderate	Severe
Salinity $EC_w{}^a$		dS/m	<0.7	0.7–3.0	>3.0
TDS		mg/l	<450	450–2000	>2000
TSS		mg/l	<50	50–100	>100
SAR[b]	0–3	meq/l	>0.7 EC_w	0.7–0.2 EC_w	<0.2 EC_w
SAR	3–6	meq/l	>1.2 EC_w	1.2–0.3 EC_w	<0.3 EC_w
SAR	6–12	meq/l	>1.9 EC_w	1.9–0.5 EC_w	<0.5 EC_w
SAR	12–20	meq/l	>2.9 EC_w	2.9–1.3 EC_w	<1.3 EC_w
SAR	20–40	meq/l	>5.0 EC_w	5.0–2.9 EC_w	<2.9 EC_w
Sodium (Na^+)	Sprinkler irrigation	meq/l	<3	>3	
Sodium (Na^+)	Surface irrigation	meq/l	<3	3–9	>9
Chloride (Cl^-)	Sprinkler irrigation	meq/l	<3	>3	
Chloride (Cl^-)	Surface irrigation	meq/l	<4	4–10	>10
Chlorine (Cl_2)	Total residual	mg/l	<1	1–5	>5
Bicarbonate ($HCO_3{}^-$)		mg/l	<90	90–500	>500
Boron (B)		mg/l	<0.7	0.7–3.0	>3.0
Hydrogen sulfide (H_2S)		mg/l	<0.5	0.5–2.0	> 2.0
Iron (Fe)	Drip irrigation	mg/l	<0.1	0.1–1.5	>1.5
Manganese (Mn)	Drip irrigation	mg/l	<0.1	0.1–1.5	>1.5
Total nitrogen (TN)		mg/l	<5	5–30	>30
pH			Normal range 6.5–8		
Trace elements (see Table A1.2)					

TDS, total dissolved solids; TSS, total suspended solids
Sources: Ayers & Westcot (1985); Pescod (1992); Asano & Levine (1998).
[a] EC_w means electrical conductivity in deciSiemens per metre at 25 °C.
[b] SAR means sodium adsorption ratio ($[meq/l]^{1/2}$); see section A1.5.

Sodium chloride, boron and selenium should be monitored carefully. Many plants are sensitive to these substances. Boron is frequently present in wastewater because it is used in household detergents. Many types of trees (e.g. citrus and stone fruits) will have impaired growth even when low boron concentrations are present in the water (Ayers & Westcot, 1985). Selenium can be toxic to plants in very low concentrations and can accumulate in plant tissue to toxic concentrations — for example, in alfalfa grown for forage (Tanji & Kielen, 2002). Concentrations of these elements in the irrigation water may be improved by blending water supplies if other water sources are available. See FAO Publication 61, chapter 6, on details regarding blending of water supplies for irrigation (Tanji & Kielen, 2002).

Water quality is also a factor in selecting the type of irrigation method. For example, sprinkler irrigation with water that contains relatively high concentrations of sodium or chloride ions can cause leaf damage to sensitive crops, especially when climatic conditions favour evaporation (i.e. high temperatures and low humidity) (Ayers & Westcot, 1985). Similar damage to crops occurs when wastewater with high levels of residual chlorine (>5 mg/l) is sprayed directly onto leaves (Asano & Levine, 1998).

Municipal wastewater may contain a range of other toxic substances, including heavy metals, as a result of industrial effluents entering the municipal wastewater stream (Pescod, 1992). Some of these substances may be removed during wastewater treatment processes when available, but others may remain in quantities large enough to cause toxicity to the crops. In cases where industrial wastes are released into the general wastewater stream or where crops exhibit signs of trace element toxicity, it may be necessary to test the water and soil for these elements. Heavy metals are usually fixed by the soil matrix and tend to be mobile only in the topmost soil layers. When water containing toxic trace elements is applied to crops, these elements may be concentrated in the soil as the water is lost into the atmosphere (Tanji & Kielen, 2002). Table A1.2 shows the threshold values for plant toxicity for selected trace elements.

Table A1.2 Threshold levels of trace elements for crop production

Element		Recommended maximum concentration[a] (mg/l)	Remarks
Al	Aluminium	5.0	Can cause non-productivity in acid soils (pH <5.5), but more alkaline soils at pH >7.0 will precipitate the ion and eliminate any toxicity.
As	Arsenic	0.10	Toxicity to plants varies widely, ranging from 12 mg/l for Sudan grass to less than 0.05 mg/l for rice.
Be	Beryllium	0.10	Toxicity to plants varies widely, ranging from 5 mg/l for kale to 0.5 mg/l for bush beans.
Cd	Cadmium	0.01	Toxic to beans, beets and turnips at concentrations as low as 0.1 mg/l in nutrient solutions. Conservative limits recommended due to its potential for accumulation in plants and soils to concentrations that may be harmful to humans.
Co	Cobalt	0.05	Toxic to tomato plants at 0.1 mg/l in nutrient solution. Tends to be inactivated by neutral and alkaline soils.
Cr	Chromium	0.10	Not generally recognized as an essential growth element. Conservative limits recommended due to lack of knowledge on its toxicity to plants.
Cu[b]	Copper	0.20	Toxic to a number of plants at 0.1–1.0 mg/l in nutrient solutions.
F	Fluoride	1.0	Inactivated by neutral and alkaline soils.
Fe[b]	Iron	5.0	Not toxic to plants in aerated soils, but can contribute to soil acidification and loss of availability of essential phosphorus and molybdenum. Overhead sprinkling may result in unsightly deposits on plants, equipment and buildings.

Table A1.2 (continued)

Element		Recommended maximum concentration[a] (mg/l)	Remarks
Li	Lithium	2.5	Tolerated by most crops up to 5 mg/l; mobile in soil. Toxic to citrus at low concentrations (<0.075 mg/l). Acts similarly to boron.
Mn[b]	Manganese	0.20	Toxic to a number of crops at a few-tenths to a few mg/l, but usually only in acid soils.
Mo	Molybdenum	0.01	Not toxic to plants at normal concentrations in soil and water. Can be toxic to livestock if forage is grown in soils with high concentrations of available molybdenum.
Ni	Nickel	0.20	Toxic to a number of plants at 0.5–1.0 mg/l; reduced toxicity at neutral or alkaline pH.
Pd	Lead	5.0	Can inhibit plant cell growth at very high concentrations.
Se	Selenium	0.02	Toxic to plants at concentrations as low as 0.025 mg/l, and toxic to livestock if forage is grown in soils with relatively high levels of added selenium. Essential element to animals, but in very low concentrations.
V	Vanadium	0.10	Toxic to many plants at relatively low concentrations.
Zn[b]	Zinc	2.0	Toxic to many plants at widely varying concentrations; reduced toxicity at pH >6.0 and in fine textured or organic soils.

Source: Adapted from Ayers & Westcot (1985); Pescod (1992).

[a] The maximum concentration is based on a water application rate that is consistent with good irrigation practices (5000–10 000 m³/ha per year). If the water application rate greatly exceeds this, the maximum concentrations should be adjusted downward accordingly. No adjustment should be made for application rates less than 10 000 m³/ha per year. The values given are for water used on a continuous basis at one site.

[b] Synergistic action of Cu and Zn and antagonistic action of Fe and Mn have been reported in certain plants species' absorption and tolerance of metals after wastewater irrigation. If the irrigation water contains high concentrations of Cu and Zn, Cu concentrations in the tissue may increase greatly. In plants irrigated with water containing a high concentration of Mn, Mn uptake in the plants may increase, and, consequently, the concentration of Fe in the plant tissue may be reduced considerably. Generally, metal concentrations in plant tissue increase with concentrations in the irrigation water. Concentrations in the roots are usually higher than in the leaves (Drakatos, Kalavrouziotis & Drakatos, 2000; Drakatos et al., 2002; Kalavrouziotis & Drakotos, 2002).

A1.4 Soil characteristics

Soil infiltration

The infiltration rate of the soil determines how much water will reach the crop root zone and eventually percolate to the subsoil and is dependent upon soil texture and structure and the structural stability of the soil. The infiltration rate is also dependent upon both the salinity of the water and the sodium adsorption ratio (SAR) of the soil (see Table A1.1). The SAR is a measure of the ratio of sodium ions to calcium and magnesium ions in the soil. The SAR can be calculated using the following formula:

$$SAR = Na^+/[(Ca^{++} + Mg^{++})/2]^{1/2}$$

where the ionic concentrations of Na, Ca and Mg are expressed in meq/l.

Water with a low salinity content (<0.5 dS/m) leaches soluble minerals and salts. If calcium is leached, soil structure can be destabilized and fine soil particles become dispersed. These fine soil particles clog the pore spaces. This leads to reduced water infiltration rates, soil crusting and crop emergence problems (Ayers & Westcot, 1985). Water with excessive sodium (relative to the concentration of total dissolved salts in the soil) also will impair water infiltration (Pescod, 1992). Water infiltration problems usually occur in the top 10 cm of the soil (Asano & Levine, 1998).

Drainage
To maintain a favourable salt balance, excess water must be able to drain from the surface and from the root zone. Excess water can damage plants and increase soil salinity. Good drainage is particularly important in arid and semi-arid areas. If land drainage is insufficient, the water table can rise. When the water table gets too close to the surface (within 2 m), during dry periods water can rise to the surface by capillary action, evaporate and leave behind dissolved salts. Salt accumulation in the soil reduces crop yields and can ultimately make the soil unfit for agriculture (Pescod, 1992). In areas where the water table is high and the groundwater has a high salinity, it may be necessary to construct open or tile drains to stabilize the depth of the groundwater (Ayers & Westcot, 1985). The long-term sustainability of irrigation with wastewater requires soils with good drainage (Asano & Levine, 1998). As the drainage water can contain components that may be harmful to the environment (e.g. salts, pesticide and fertilizer residues), the quality of the drainage water should be controlled and must be disposed of properly, particularly if it is reused in agriculture or for other purposes. (Tanji & Kielen, 2002). Wescot (1997) describes quality characteristics of drainage water from agriculture.

A1.5 Crop selection
Crops vary by as much as 10-fold in their ability to tolerate salt. In situations where soil salinity is high or the irrigation water (wastewater in this case) has a salinity above 3 dS/m, it may be necessary to grow more salt-tolerant crops (Pescod, 1992). Another alternative may be to adopt an integrated farm drainage management approach. Under such an approach, water is used sequentially to irrigate crops, trees and halophytes with progressively increasing salt tolerance (Tanji & Kielen, 2002). Comprehensive information on crops and their salt tolerances is given in FAO Publications 29, 47 and 61 (Ayers & Westcot, 1985; Pescod, 1992; Tanji & Kielen, 2002).

A1.6 Leaching
One of the most important water quality parameters for irrigation is salinity. Excess salinity can alter soil properties and damage plants or reduce crop yields (Asano & Levine, 1998). Wastewater that has too much salinity (measured as total dissolved solids, or TDS; see Table A1.1) may cause salt to build up to excessive levels in the crop root zone. One way to control salinity problems is to apply enough water to ensure that the salts are carried below the root zone. This is called leaching. For irrigation to be sustainable over a long period of time, the soil must have good drainage properties. To ensure that salts move downwards from the upper root zone through the lower root zone, sufficient leaching must take place. The proportion of irrigation water that passes through the entire root zone is called the leaching fraction (LF) (Asano & Levine, 1998).

LF =   depth of water leached below the root zone / depth of water applied at the surface

The salt concentration in the root zone is inversely proportional to LF. For irrigation with wastewater, it is best to have LF >0.5 (for heavy clay soils, this number will be >0.1). In cases where the salinity of the irrigation water and LF are known, the salinity of the drainage water below the root zone can be predicted from the following equation (Asano & Levine, 1998):

$$EC_{DW} = EC_W/LF$$

where EC_{DW} and EC_W are the electrical conductivities of the drainage water and the irrigation water, respectively.

A1.7 Management practices

Good management practices are important in any irrigation scheme. In addition to those practices previously described for controlling health impacts, it is also necessary for optimal plant growth to properly manage water application rates and timing, land and soil and crops. A summary of these considerations is presented below. More detailed information on irrigation management strategies is given in Pescod (1992) and Ayers & Westcot (1985).

It is necessary to manage water application rates and to time applications appropriately. It is important to:

- assess the water-holding capacity of the soil;
- assess the need for pre- and post-planting irrigation to avoid water stress and leach salts from soil prior to and after planting;
- maintain optimal soil moisture levels;
- estimate the evapotranspiration rate (mostly based on the prevailing climatic conditions — e.g. radiation, temperature, humidity and wind speed);
- time water applications appropriately — e.g. water can be applied at night to reduce losses to evaporation and reduce sodium and chloride toxicity to plants;
- determine the quantity of water to be applied, based on rainfall, drainage, soil infiltration, plant and leaching requirements;
- adjust the nitrogen level to match plant requirements through water blending;
- evaluate the irrigation method (e.g. water with residual chlorine applied via sprinkler irrigation can harm the leaves of many plants);
- assess soil drainage properties.

Land and soil management are important for overcoming salinity, sodicity (sodium concentration in the soil) and toxicity to plants and reducing health hazards. The following practices need to be considered to optimize plant growth in specific conditions:

- grading the land to reduce erosion and runoff;
- deep ploughing to break up compact soil pans and improve water movement through the soil;
- soil amendments to improve soil structure, drainage, infiltration or pH.

Crop management can also be used to improve yields. Irrigation with wastewater may require management practices similar to those for irrigation with saline water. Seed germination is most sensitive to soil salinity. Seeds can be placed in such a way as to minimize the impacts of soil salinity by:

- crop selection according to salt tolerance;
- planting seeds on the shoulder(s) of the ridge during furrow irrigation;
- planting seeds on the sloping side of seed beds (seeds should be placed above the water line);
- irrigating alternate rows so that salts move beyond the single seed row;
- choosing alternatives to furrow irrigation when the wastewater is highly saline.

A1.9 Conclusion

Once the barriers for health protection are put into place, the use of wastewater in agriculture requires many of the management practices used for irrigation with any type of water. Special attention needs to be given to water quality (contents of salts, nutrients and toxic trace elements), as these may have an impact on crop growth, yield and soil properties. Several FAO Irrigation and Drainage Papers and Water Reports provide more detailed information on good irrigation and drainage practices.

A1.10 References[1]

Allen RG et al. (1998). *Crop evapotranspiration — Guidelines for computing crop water requirements.* Rome, Food and Agriculture Organization of the United Nations (FAO Irrigation and Drainage Paper 56).

Asano T, Levine AD (1998). Wastewater reclamation, recycling, and reuse: an introduction. In: Asano T, ed. *Wastewater reclamation and reuse.* Lancaster, PA, Technomic Publishing Company, pp. 1–56.

Ayers RS, Westcot DW (1985) *Water quality for agriculture.* Rome, Food and Agriculture Organization of the United Nations (FAO Irrigation and Drainage Paper 29, Revision 1; http://www.fao.org/docrep/003/T0234E/T0234E00.htm).

Drakatos PA, Kalavrouziotis IK, Drakatos SP (2000). Synergism of Cu and Zn in the plants irrigated via processed liquid wastewater. *Journal of Land Contamination and Reclamation*, 8(3):201–207.

Drakatos PA et al. (2002). Antagonistic action of Fe and Mn in Mediterranean-type plants irrigated with wastewater effluents following biological treatment. *International Journal of Environmental Studies*, 59(1):125–132.

Kalavrouziotis IK, Drakatos PA (2002). Irrigation of certain Mediterranean plants with heavy metals. *International Journal of Environment and Pollution*, 18(3):294–300.

Pescod MB (1992). *Wastewater treatment and use in agriculture.* Rome, Food and Agriculture Organization of the United Nations (FAO Irrigation and Drainage Paper 47).

Tanji KK, Kielen NC (2002). *Agricultural drainage water management in arid and semi-arid areas.* Rome, Food and Agriculture Organization of the United Nations (FAO Irrigation and Drainage Paper 61).

Westcot DW (1997). *Drainage water quality.* In: Madramootoo CA, Johnston WR, Williardson LS, eds. *Management of agricultural drainage water quality.* Rome, Food and Agriculture Organization of the United Nations (Water Report 13).

---

[1] Most FAO publications can be found online at http://www.fao.org/documents/ or http://www.fao.org/ag/agl/public.stm.

Summary of impacts of heavy metals and trace elements associated with wastewater irrigation

Table A2.1: Summary of studies that analyse the effects of metals in wastewater irrigation

Description of the study	Type of study			References
	In field	Demonstration projects	Laboratory study	
Sewage				
In San Angelo, Texas, USA, the long-term application of treated wastewater to forage grasses did not increase the Cd, Cu or Zn content above regional background values. Only Cr and Ni displayed high concentrations, but without exceeding guidelines.	X			Hossner, Kao & Waggoner (1978)
In Dickinson, North Dakota, USA, a long-term effects study found, in forage grasses watered with treated wastewater, a 28% increase in B, a 47% increase in Mn and a 68% increase in Zn levels without exceeding the permissible limits. Cd, Cr, Co, Pb and Mo did not show any change, while Cu diminished by 8%.	X			Benham-Blair & Affiliates, Inc. & Engineering Enterprises, Inc. (1979)
Long-term irrigation with reclaimed water in the USA did not produce negative effects in tomatoes, broccoli, forage grasses, grain corn, barley, alfalfa sorghum, pasture, beans, carrots, lettuce, peas, radishes, sweet corn and wheat.	X			USEPA (1981)
In an overflow soil aquifer treatment system in Mississippi, USA, no adverse effects were observed in grasses. Metal accumulation was higher near the site of the application of the wastewater (uphill) and decreased with distance down the treatment slope. Grass uptake accounted only for 1.2, 1.4, 4.0 and 7.6% of the applied Cd, Ni, Cu and Zn, respectively.	X			Peters, Lee & Bates (1980)
In Melbourne, Australia, irrigation for 76 years with treated wastewaters showed no significant accumulation of Cd in soils and plants in comparison with sites receiving fresh water.	X			Metcalf & Eddy, Inc. (1991)
In Isfahan, Iran, the use of wastewater in agriculture for eight years did not significantly increase Zn, Mg, Cu or Fe levels in soil (up to 40 cm depth). However, the contents of these metals in corn, wheat and tomato were significantly higher than those in crops irrigated with well water, although the United States Environmental Protection Agency guidelines were not surpassed in any case.	X			Feizi (2001)
Metal content in municipal wastewaters has not presented difficulties for irrigation in Australia, unless a local metal industry discharges effluents to the sewerage system.	X			AATSE (2004)
In Haroonabad, India, irrigation with domestic wastewater for 35 years has caused a significant accumulation of Pb and Cu within the top 0–15 cm of soil (9 vs 8 mg Pb/kg and 87 vs 22 mg Cu/kg), but not of Zn, Co, Cr and Mn. Despite this, all heavy metal concentrations in soils were within European Economic Community maximum permissible levels. At the current rate of	X			

Table A2.1 (continued)

Description of the study	Type of study			References
	In field	Demonstration projects	Laboratory study	
accumulation, metals will not prove to be a risk in the coming decades, although strategic monitoring is recommended.				
A comparison of metal absorption in different crops watered with sewage, a 50% dilution with fresh water and fresh water only showed that the amount of metals absorbed depended on the type of crops and not only on the metal concentration in water; metal absorption was not necessarily greater when using sewage.			X	Simmons & Pongaskul (2002)
Irrigation with wastewater for more than 80 years in the Mezquital Valley, Mexico, has increased the original metal content in soils by 3–6 times, but concentrations are still below international criteria. Contamination has not been reported in crops. Metals were found to be bound to soil due to its organic matter content.	X			Siebe & Fischer (1996)
Type of wastewater not specified				
Soils having about 0.4–0.5 mg Cd/kg produced brown rice with 0.08 mg Cd/kg; and soils with a content of 0.82–2.1 mg Cd/kg produced heavily contaminated brown rice (1 mg Cd/kg).		X		Morishita (1988)
Wastewaters with industrial influence				
In the Bahr Bagar Drain in Egypt, which is used for irrigation, 75% of the flow is wastewater. Irrigated soils contain 5 mg Cd/kg, which is double the original value. There is evidence that Cd is being absorbed by crops. The Cd content in rice is 1.6 mg/kg.	X			FAO (2003)
Industrial wastewaters				
Reed canary-grass and maize were irrigated for six years with an effluent containing Cu, Cd, Pb and Zn without creating health problems. Nevertheless, when sludge was added in addition to wastewater for seven years, the Cu was thought to pose a risk to sheep fed with these crops. It was determined that crop removal in areas where heavy metal application was low could possibly increase the disposal life of the site.		X		Sidle, Hook & Kardos (1976)
A textile industry effluent diluted with fresh water used to irrigate rice, kidney beans and lady's fingers increased productivity due to its organic matter content up to a 75% effluent; beyond this dilution, effluent inhibited growth.		X		Ajmal & Khan (1985)
In India, an effluent from a paper mill industry was used to irrigate coconut trees. It was found that the Cu, Pb, Zn, Co and Cd content exceeded Codex Alimentarius Commission guidelines in crops.			X	Fazel et al. (1991)

Table A2.1 (continued)

Description of the study	Type of study			References
	In field	**Demonstration projects**	**Laboratory study**	
A paper industry effluent was used with different dilutions of fresh water to irrigate rice. As the proportion of effluent increased, the quality of germination, the growth rate and the pigments were negatively impacted.		X		Misra & Behera (1991)
An oil refinery treated effluent was used to irrigate four varieties of wheat for eight years. Fresh water was used as a control. Productivity was found to increase, so it was recommended that the metal content be periodically monitored to avoid possible risks.		X		Aziz et al. (1996)
An effluent spiked with Cd, Cr and Pb (up to 100 mg/l) was used to irrigate soils at different pH values (including acid ones), soil grain size (<180–2000 μm), TOC content in solution (0 and 6.3 mg C/l) and water flow (0.3 and 0.7 m^3/m^2 per hour). All the metals were quickly adsorbed in soils, even at pH 4.3. Metal concentration in wastewater was found to be the variable that most determined adsorption.			X	Lee et al. (2004)

A2.1 References

AATSE (2004). *Water recycling in Australia.* Melbourne, Australian Academy of Technological Sciences and Engineering.

Ajmal M, Khan AU (1985). Effect of textile factory effluent on soil and crop plants. *Environmental Pollution,* 37:131–148.

Aziz O et al. (1996). Long-term effects of irrigation with petrochemical industry wastewater. *Journal of Environmental Science and Health,* 31(10):2595–2620.

Benham-Blair & Affiliates, Inc., Engineering Enterprises, Inc. (1979). *Long-term effects of land application of domestic wastewater. Dickinson, North Dakota, slow rate irrigation site.* Washington, DC, United States Environmental Protection Agency (EPA-600/2-79-144).

FAO (2003). *Unlocking water potential in agriculture.* Rome, Food and Agriculture Organization of the United Nations (http://www.fao.org/documents/show_cdr.asp?url_file=/DOCREP/006/Y4525E/Y4525E00.HTM).

Fazel M et al. (1991). Effect of paper mill effluents on accumulation of heavy metals in coconut trees near Nanjangud, Mysore District, Karnataka, India. *Environmental Geology and Water Science,* 17(1):47–50.

Feizi M (2001). Effect of treated wastewater on accumulation of heavy metals in plants and soil. In: *Proceedings of the first Asian Regional Conference of ICID, Seoul, Korea.* New Delhi, International Commission on Irrigation and Drainage.

Hossner LR, Kao CW, Waggoner JA (1978). *Sewage disposal on agricultural soils; chemical and microbiological implications.* Washington, DC, United States Environmental Protection Agency (EPA-600/s-78-131a).

Lee S et al. (2004). Sorption behaviors of heavy metals in SAT (soil aquifer treatment) system. *Water Science and Technology,* 50(2):263–268.

Matsuno Y et al. (2004). Assessment of the use of wastewater for irrigation: a case in Punjab, Pakistan. In: Steenvoorden J, Endreny T, eds. *Wastewater re-use and groundwater quality.* Wallingford, International Association of Hydrological Sciences (IAHS Publication 285).

Metcalf & Eddy, Inc. (1991). *Wastewater: treatment, reuse and disposal.* New York, McGraw-Hill.

Misra R, Behera P (1991). The effect of paper industry effluent on growth, pigment, carbohydrate and protein of rice seedlings. *Environmental Pollution,* 72:159–167.

Morishita T (1988). Environmental hazards of sewage and industrial effluents on irrigated farmlands in Japan. In: Pescod MB, Arar A, eds. *Treatment and use of sewage effluent for irrigation.* Kent, Butterworths.

Peters R, Lee C, Bates D (1980). *Field investigations of overland flow treatment of municipal lagoon effluent.* Vicksburg, MS, United States Army Corps of Engineers, Waterways Experiment Station.

Sidle RC, Hook JE, Kardos LT (1976). Heavy metal application and plant uptake in a land disposal system for wastewater. *Journal of Environmental Quality,* 5(1):97–102.

Siebe C, Fischer W (1996). Effect of long term irrigation with untreated sewage effluents on soil properties and heavy metals absorption of leptosols and vertisols in Central Mexico. *Pflanzenernahrsm Bodenk,* 159:357–364.

Simmons RW, Pongsakul P (2002). Toward the development of an effective sampling protocol to "rapidly" evaluate the distribution of Cd in contaminated, irrigated rice-based agricultural systems. In: Kheoruenromne I, ed. *Transactions of the 17th world congress of soil science, Bangkok, 14–21 August 2002.* Vienna, International Union of Soil Science.

USEPA (1981). *Land treatment of municipal wastewater.* Washington, DC, United States Environmental Protection Agency (EPA 625/1-81/013).

Health impact assessment

Health impact assessment (HIA) is an instrument for safeguarding the health of vulnerable communities in the context of accelerated changes in environmental and/or social health determinants resulting from development. WHO/ECHP (1999) defined HIA as "A combination of procedures, methods and tools by which a policy, programme or project may be judged as to its potential effects on the health of a population, and the distribution of those effects within the population." A health impact is a change in health risk reasonably attributable to a project, programme or policy. A health risk is the likelihood of a health hazard affecting a particular community at a particular time. Assessments can be retrospective or prospective. Retrospective assessments measure and record what has happened, while prospective assessments facilitate development planning and help to predict the consequences of a future project based on available evidence (WHO, 2000).

A3.1 Procedures and methods
In Figure A3.1, the sequence of essential HIA procedures is presented, with an indication of when each method is applied. Effective HIA requires health hazards, risks, determinants and potential impacts to be defined and monitored (WHO, 2001). Implementation of these procedures should be done in such a way that all relevant stakeholders are involved — especially the local communities that will be impacted.

Figure A3.1

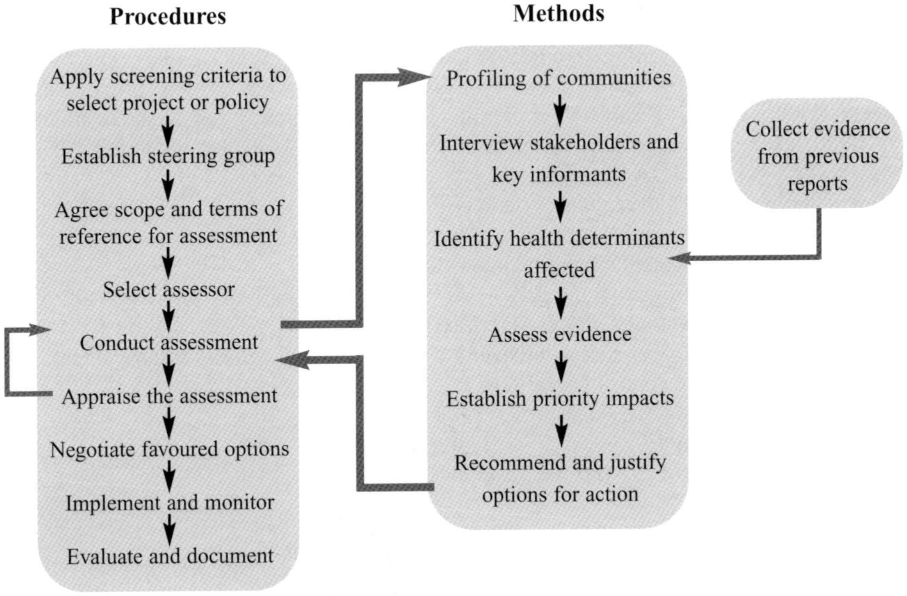

Procedures and methods of HIA (WHO, 2000)

When policy and procedure have been established, the actual assessment can take place. It consists of inferring changes in health determinants that are reasonably attributable to the project and that could affect each stakeholder community during each stage of the project. The changes, taken together, produce health outcomes or changes in health status. These are expressed in a minimum of three ranks: no change, increased health risk and increased health enhancement. Quantification is generally difficult, either because the data are lacking or because there are no known functional relationships between cause and effect. Research is needed to improve the predictive models for other health concerns.

The best forecast of what will happen is the history of what has happened with similar wastewater-based agricultural activities in comparable regions (WHO, 2000).

The assessment would start by collecting baseline data on wastewater use in agriculture and health risks over a period of at least two years prior to final agreement on project design. This will provide a profile of the existing communities, their environment, seasonal changes in health risks and the capabilities of their institutions. The data collection would be repeated after the project was operational, and the difference would provide a record of health impact and its likely causes. The record would add to the available knowledge base and improve the assessment of future projects.

The objective of HIA is to present evidence, infer changes and recommend actions to safeguard, mitigate and enhance human health. The inferences may not always be founded on extensive data, but they must be persuasive (WHO, 2000).

A3.2 Management of health risks and enhancements

The final stage of the assessment is to recommend and budget socially acceptable measures to safeguard, mitigate and promote human health (WHO, 2000). The most important principle for health promotion is dialogue between project proponents, health professionals and stakeholder communities at the planning stage. The technical recommendations for managing health risks are diverse. A broad classification is:

- appropriate health regulations and enforcement;
- modifications to project plans and operations;
- improved management and maintenance;
- supportive infrastructure, such as the installation or improvement of wastewater treatment and use facilities;
- timely provision of accessible health care, including diagnosis and treatment;
- special disease control operations;
- individual protective measures;
- health education;
- redistribution of risk through insurance schemes.

A3.3 References

WHO (2000). *Human health and dams, the World Health Organization's submission to the World Commission on Dams (WCD)*. Geneva, World Health Organization (Document WHO/SDE/WSH/00.01).

WHO (2001). *Health impact assessment (HIA), report of an inter-regional meeting on harmonization and mainstreaming of HIA in the World Health Organization and of a partnership meeting on the institutionalization of HIA capacity building in Africa, Arusha, 31 October – 3 November 2000*. Geneva, World Health Organization.

WHO/ECHP (1999). *Gothenburg consensus paper, 1999 — Health impact assessment: main concepts and suggested approach*. Brussels, European Centre for Health Policy, World Health Organization Regional Office for Europe (http://www.phel.gov.uk/hiadocs/Gothenburgpaper.pdf).

Annex 4
Glossary of terms used in the Guidelines

This glossary does not aim to provide precise definitions of technical or scientific terms, but rather to explain in plain language the meaning of terms frequently used in these Guidelines.

Abattoir – Slaughterhouse where animals are killed and processed into food and other products.

Advanced or tertiary treatment – Treatment steps added after the secondary treatment stage to remove specific constituents, such as nutrients, suspended solids, organics, heavy metals or dissolved solids (e.g. salts).

Anaerobic pond – Treatment pond where anaerobic digestion and sedimentation of organic wastes occur; usually the first type of pond in a waste stabilization pond system; requires periodic removal of accumulated sludge formed as a result of sedimentation.

Aquaculture – Raising plants or animals in water (water farming).

Aquifer – A geological area that produces a quantity of water from permeable rock.

Arithmetic mean – The sum of the values of all samples divided by the number of samples; provides the average number per sample.

Biochemical oxygen demand (BOD) – The amount of oxygen that is required to biochemically convert organic matter into inert substances; an indirect measure of the amount of biodegradable organic matter present in the water or wastewater.

Buffer zone – Land that separates wastewater, excreta and/or greywater use areas from public access areas; used to prevent exposures to the public from hazards associated with wastewater, excreta and/or greywater.

Cartage – The process of manually transporting faecal material off site for disposal or treatment.

Coagulation – The clumping together of particles to increase the rate at which sedimentation occurs. Usually triggered by the addition of certain chemicals (e.g. lime, aluminium sulfate, ferric chloride).

Constructed wetlands – Engineered pond or tank-type units to treat faecal sludge or wastewater; consist of a filtering body planted with aquatic emergent plants.

Cost–benefit analysis – An analysis of all the costs of a project and all of the benefits. Projects that provide the most benefits at the least cost are the most desirable.

Cyst – Environmentally resistant infective parasitic life stage (e.g. *Giardia*, *Taenia*).

Cysticercosis – Infection with *Taenia solium* (pig tapeworm) sometimes leads to cysticerci (an infective life stage) encysting in the brain of humans, leading to neurological symptoms such as epilepsy.

Depuration – Transfer of fish to clean water prior to consumption in an attempt to purge their bodies of contamination, potentially including some pathogenic microorganisms.

Diarrhoea – Loose, watery and frequent bowel movements, often associated with an infection.

Disability adjusted life years (DALYs) – Population metric of life years lost to disease due to both morbidity and mortality.

Disease – Symptoms of illness in a host, e.g. diarrhoea, fever, vomiting, blood in urine, etc.

Disinfection – The inactivation of pathogenic organisms using chemicals, radiation, heat or physical separation processes (e.g. membranes).

Drain – A conduit or channel constructed to carry off stormwater runoff, wastewater or other surplus water. Drains can be open ditches or lined, unlined or buried pipes.

Drip irrigation – Irrigation delivery systems that deliver drips of water directly to plants through pipes. Small holes or emitters control the amount of water that is released to the plant. Drip irrigation does not contaminate aboveground plant surfaces.

Dual-media filtration – Filtration technique that uses two types of filter media to remove particulate matter with different chemical and physical properties (e.g. sand, anthracite, diatomaceous earth).

Effluent – Liquid (e.g. treated or untreated wastewater) that flows out of a process or confined space).

Encyst – The development of a protective cyst for the infective stage of different parasites (e.g. helminths such as foodborne trematodes, tapeworms, and some protozoa such as *Giardia*).

Epidemiology – The study of the distribution and determinants of health-related states or events in specified populations, and the application of this study to the control of health problems.

***Escherichia coli* (*E. coli*)** – A bacterium found in the gut, used as an indicator of faecal contamination of water.

Excreta – Faeces and urine (see also faecal sludge, septage and nightsoil).

Exposure – Contact of a chemical, physical or biological agent with the outer boundary of an organism (e.g. through inhalation, ingestion or dermal contact).

Exposure assessment – The estimation (qualitative or quantitative) of the magnitude, frequency, duration, route and extent of exposure to one or more contaminated media.

Facultative pond – Aerobic pond used to degrade organic matter and inactivate pathogens; usually the second type of pond in a waste stabilization pond system.

Faecal sludge – Sludges of variable consistency collected from on-site sanitation systems, such as latrines, non-sewered public toilets, septic tanks and aqua privies. Septage, the faecal sludge collected from septic tanks, is included in this term (see also excreta and nightsoil).

Flocculation – The agglomeration of colloidal and finely divided suspended matter after coagulation by gentle stirring by either mechanical or hydraulic means.

Geometric mean – A measure of central tendency, just like a median. It is different from the traditional mean (which is called the arithmetic mean) because it uses multiplication rather than addition to summarize data values. The geometric mean is a useful summary when changes in the data occur in a relative fashion.

Greywater – Water from the kitchen, bath and/or laundry, which generally does not contain significant concentrations of excreta.

Groundwater – Water contained in rocks or subsoil.

Grow-out pond – Pond used to raise adult fish from fingerlings.

Hazard – A biological, chemical, physical or radiological agent that has the potential to cause harm.

Health-based target – A defined level of health protection for a given exposure. This can be based on a measure of disease, e.g. 10^{-6} DALY per person per year, or the absence of a specific disease related to that exposure.

Health impact assessment – The estimation of the effects of any specific action (plans, policies or programmes) in any given environment on the health of a defined population.

High-growing crops – Crops that grow above the ground and do not normally touch it (e.g. fruit trees).

High-rate treatment processes – Engineered treatment processes characterized by high flow rates and low hydraulic retention times. Usually include a primary treatment step to settle solids followed by a secondary treatment step to biodegrade organic substances.

Hydraulic retention time – Time the wastewater takes to pass through the system.

Hypochlorite – Chemical frequently used for disinfection (sodium or calcium hypochlorite).

Indicator organisms – Microorganisms whose presence is indicative of faecal contamination and possibly of the presence of more harmful microorganisms.

Infection – The entry and development or multiplication of an infectious agent in a host. Infection may or may not lead to disease symptoms (e.g. diarrhoea). Infection can be measured by detecting infectious agents in excreta or colonized areas or through measurement of a host immune response (i.e. the presence of antibodies against the infectious agent).

Intermediate host – The host occupied by juvenile stages of a parasite prior to the definitive host and in which asexual reproduction often occurs (e.g. for foodborne trematodes or schistosomes the intermediate hosts are specific species of snails).

Legislation – Law enacted by a legislative body or the act of making or enacting laws.

Localized irrigation – Irrigation application technologies that apply the water directly to the crop, either through drip irrigation or bubbler irrigation. Generally use less water and result in less crop contamination and reduce human contact with the wastewater.

Log reduction – Organism removal efficiencies: 1 log unit = 90%; 2 log units = 99%; 3 log units = 99.9%; and so on.

Low-growing crops – Crops that grow below, on or near the soil surface (e.g. carrots, lettuce).

Low-rate biological treatment systems – Use biological processes to treat wastewater in large basins, usually earthen ponds. Characterized by long hydraulic retention times. Examples of low-rate biological treatment processes include waste stabilization ponds, wastewater storage and treatment reservoirs and constructed wetlands.

Maturation pond – An aerobic pond with algal growth and high levels of bacterial removal; usually the final type of pond in a waste stabilization pond system.

Median – The middle value of a sample series (50% of the values in the sample are lower and 50% are greater than the median).

Membrane filtration – Filtration technique based on a physical barrier (a membrane) with specific pore sizes that traps contaminants larger than the pore size on the top surface of the membrane. Contaminants smaller than the specified pore size may pass through the membrane or may be captured within the membrane by some other mechanism.

Metacercariae (infective) – Life cycle stage of trematode parasites infective to humans. Metacercariae can form cysts in fish muscle tissue or on the surfaces of plants, depending on the type of trematode species.

Multiple barriers – Use of more than one preventive measure as a barrier against hazards.

Nightsoil – Untreated excreta transported without water, e.g. via containers or buckets; often used as a popular term in an unspecific manner to designate faecal matter of any origin; its technical use is therefore not recommended.

Off-site sanitation – System of sanitation where excreta are removed from the plot occupied by the dwelling and its immediate surroundings.

On-site sanitation – System of sanitation where the means of storage are contained within the plot occupied by the dwelling and its immediate surroundings. For some systems (e.g. double-pit or vault latrines), treatment of the faecal matter happens on site also, through extended in-pit consolidation and storage. With other systems (e.g. septic tanks, single-pit or vault installations), the sludge has to be collected and treated off site (see also faecal sludge).

Oocyst – A structure that is produced by some coccidian protozoa (i.e. *Cryptosporidium*) as a result of sexual reproduction during the life cycle. The oocyst is usually the infectious and environmental stage, and it contains sporozoites. For the enteric protozoa, the oocyst is excreted in the faeces.

Operational monitoring – The act of conducting a planned sequence of observations or measurements of control parameters to assess whether a control measure is operating within design specifications (e.g. for wastewater treatment turbidity). Emphasis is given to monitoring parameters that can be measured quickly and easily and that can indicate if a process is functioning properly. Operational monitoring data should help managers to make corrections that can prevent hazard break-through.

Overhanging latrine – A latrine that empties directly into a pond or other water body.

Pathogen – A disease-causing organism (e.g. bacteria, helminths, protozoa and viruses).

pH – An expression of the intensity of the basic or acid condition of a liquid.

Policy – The set of procedures, rules and allocation mechanisms that provide the basis for programmes and services. Policies set priorities and often allocate resources for their implementation. Policies are implemented through four types of policy instruments: laws and regulations; economic measures; information and education programmes; and assignment of rights and responsibilities for providing services.

Primary treatment – Initial treatment process used to remove settleable organic and inorganic solids by sedimentation and floating substances (scum) by skimming. Examples of primary treatment include primary sedimentation, chemically enhanced primary sedimentation and upflow anaerobic sludge blanket reactors.

Quantitative microbial risk assessment (QMRA) – Method for assessing risk from specific hazards through different exposure pathways. QMRA has four components: hazard identification; exposure assessment; dose–response assessment; and risk characterization.

Regulations – Rules created by an administrative agency or body that interpret the statute(s) setting out the agency's purpose and powers or the circumstances of applying the statute.

Restricted irrigation – Use of wastewater to grow crops that are not eaten raw by humans.

Risk – The likelihood of a hazard causing harm in exposed populations in a specified time frame, including the magnitude of that harm.

Risk assessment – The overall process of using available information to predict how often hazards or specified events may occur (likelihood) and the magnitude of their consequences.

Risk management – The systematic evaluation of the wastewater, excreta or greywater use system, the identification of hazards and hazardous events, the assessment of risks and the development and implementation of preventive strategies to manage the risks.

Secondary treatment – Wastewater treatment step that follows primary treatment. Involves the removal of biodegradable dissolved and colloidal organic matter using high-rate, engineered aerobic biological treatment processes. Examples of secondary treatment include activated sludge, trickling filters, aerated lagoons and oxidation ditches.

Septage – Sludge removed from septic tanks.

Septic tank – An underground tank that treats wastewater by a combination of solids settling and anaerobic digestion. The effluents may be discharged into soak pits or small-bore sewers.

Sewage – Mixture of human excreta and water used to flush the excreta from the toilet and through the pipes; may also contain water used for domestic purposes.

Sewer – A pipe or conduit that carries wastewater or drainage water.

Sewerage – A complete system of piping, pumps, basins, tanks, unit processes and infrastructure for the collection, transporting, treating and discharging of wastewater.

Sludge – A mixture of solids and water that settles to the bottom of latrines, septic tanks and ponds or is produced as a by-product of wastewater treatment (sludge produced from the treatment of municipal or industrial wastewater is not discussed in this document).

Source separation – Diversion of urine, faeces, greywater or all, followed by separate collection (and treatment).

Subsurface irrigation – Irrigation below the soil surface; prevents contamination of aboveground parts of crops

Surface water – All water naturally open to the atmosphere (e.g. rivers, streams, lakes and reservoirs).

Thermotolerant coliforms – Group of bacteria whose presence in the environment usually indicates faecal contamination; previously called faecal coliforms.

Tolerable daily intake (TDI) – Amount of toxic substance that can be taken on a daily basis over a lifetime without exceeding a certain level of risk

Tolerable health risk – Defined level of health risk from a specific exposure or disease that is tolerated by society, used to set health-based targets.

Transmissivity – Flow capacity of an aquifer measured in volume per unit time per unit width – soil transmissivity refers to the percolation capacity of the soil.

Turbidity – The cloudiness of water caused by the presence of fine suspended matter.

Ultraviolet radiation (UV) – Light waves shorter than visible blue-violet waves of the spectrum (from 380 to 10 nanometres) used for pathogen inactivation (bacteria, protozoa and viruses).

Unrestricted irrigation – The use of treated wastewater to grow crops that are normally eaten raw.

Upflow anaerobic sludge blanket reactor – High-rate anaerobic unit used for the primary treatment of domestic wastewater. Wastewater is treated during its passage through a sludge layer (the sludge "blanket") composed of anaerobic bacteria. The treatment process is designed primarily for the removal of organic matter (biochemical oxygen demand).

Validation – Testing the system and its individual components to prove that it is capable of meeting the specified targets (i.e. microbial reduction targets). Should take place when a new system is developed or new processes are added.

Vector – Insect that carries disease from one animal or human to another (e.g. mosquitoes).

Vector-borne disease – Diseases that can be transmitted from human to human via insects (e.g. malaria).

Verification monitoring – The application of methods, procedures, tests and other evaluations, in addition to those used in operational monitoring, to determine compliance with the system design parameters and/or whether the system meets specified requirements (e.g. microbial water quality testing for *E. coli* or helminth eggs, microbial or chemical analysis of irrigated crops).

Waste-fed aquaculture – Use of wastewater, excreta and/or greywater as inputs to aquacultural systems.

Waste stabilization ponds (WSP) – Shallow basins that use natural factors such as sunlight, temperature, sedimentation, biodegradation, etc., to treat wastewater or faecal sludges. Waste stabilization pond treatment systems usually consist of anaerobic, facultative and maturation ponds linked in series.

Wastewater – Liquid waste discharged from homes, commercial premises and similar sources to individual disposal systems or to municipal sewer pipes, and which contains mainly human excreta and used water. When produced mainly by household and commercial activities, it is called domestic or municipal wastewater or domestic sewage. In this context, domestic sewage does not contain industrial effluents at levels that could pose threats to the functioning of the sewerage system, treatment plant, public health or the environment.

Withholding period – Time to allow pathogen die-off between waste application and harvest.